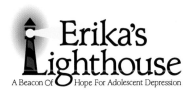

Erika's Lighthouse

A Beacon Of Hope For Adolescent Depression

PARENT HANDBOOK ON
**CHILDHOOD AND ADOLESCENT
DEPRESSION**

w: *www.erikaslighthouse.org*
e: *info@erikaslighthouse.org*

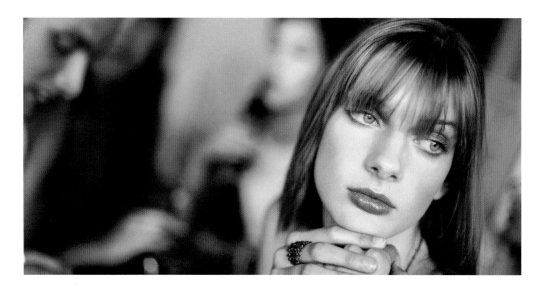

Erika's Lighthouse is a not-for-profit organization dedicated to raising awareness about childhood and adolescent depression and mental health. For more information, please visit us at *www.erikaslighthouse.org*.

PARENT HANDBOOK ON CHILDHOOD AND ADOLESCENT DEPRESSION
ISBN # 978-0-578-00976-6

The photography in this handbook is being used for illustrative purposes only; any person depicted in the photography is a model.

This handbook is based on the experiences of parents dealing with childhood and adolescent depression. It was written for parents who are in similar situations. While Erika's Lighthouse consulted with clinical, therapeutic, legal and child development experts when developing this material, it makes no representations about the medical or psychological opinions expressed herein, nor does it accept responsibility for any actions taken as a result of the material or information contained in the handbook. Every child's and family's situation is unique, and Erika's Lighthouse urges parents to seek and find competent professional advice tailored to their own family's situation. Printed in the United States

INTRODUCTION 2

SECTION ONE: A PRACTICAL GUIDE
    CHAPTER ONE: a few facts about depression 4
    CHAPTER TWO: getting help
        where to begin 7
        finding the right help 11
        getting treatment 16
    CHAPTER THREE: at home
        talking to your child 25
        talking to your family 28
        taking care of yourself 30
        one final thought 32
    CHAPTER FOUR: at school
        talking to the school 33
        getting help from the school 35
        privacy and school records 40
    CHAPTER FIVE: insurance 42

SECTION TWO: A PRIMER
    CHAPTER ONE: definitions and symptoms 45
    CHAPTER TWO: therapists 53
    CHAPTER THREE: talk therapy 57
    CHAPTER FOUR: medications 61
    CHAPTER FIVE: other treatments 74

happiness 79

a concluding letter 81

APPENDIX: a listing of mental health social service agencies
    and clinics in the northern suburbs of Chicago 82

REFERENCES AND FURTHER READING 84

SECTION ONE: A PRACTICAL GUIDE

a few facts about depression **page 4**

getting help **page 7**

at home **page 25**

at school **page 33**

insurance **page 42**

SECTION TWO: A PRIMER

definitions and symptoms **page 45**

therapists **page 53**

talk therapy **page 57**

medications **page 61**

other treatments **page 74**

Welcome to the *Erika's Lighthouse Parent Handbook on Childhood and Adolescent Depression.*

You may be reading our handbook because you think your child is depressed and you want to know what to do. **We are here to help you.**

you are
not alone

Somewhere between 15 and 20 percent of our youth will suffer from at least one depressive episode before they reach adulthood. These episodes come in many forms—ranging from the child who doesn't want to go to school to the teenager who is constantly in a rage to the withdrawn child who barely speaks.

Often, these episodes are seen as just a phase, or typical teenage behavior, but depression, clinical depression, is not part of typical teenage behavior—it is an illness that deserves attention and needs treatment.

Most children and adolescents who suffer from depression go undiagnosed and untreated. Many parents don't know the signs of depression or where to turn for help, and, if they reach out for help, they often become frustrated trying to find it. Understanding exactly what's going on with your child, finding the right treatment, dealing with the schools, negotiating insurance issues—all have their unique challenges and can deplete the energy of even the most dedicated parent.

We hope this handbook will be a helpful guide to you as you deal with the many issues you will likely confront over the course of your child's depression. We know this is probably a frightening time—many of us have been through similar times. You may feel helpless and alone. We invite you to read our handbook with the hope that it will give you both some comfort and some answers.

Please keep in mind—this is a parent-to-parent guide. It was written by parents, not professionals, and errs on the side of practical, rather than professional, advice. It is not a substitute for professional help, which we strongly encourage you to seek. And, of course, we don't have all the solutions. We merely hope that we have at least a few suggestions that will be of some practical help to you.

OUR HANDBOOK IS ORGANIZED INTO TWO SECTIONS

Section One is the practical guide—it will give you suggestions on what to do and how to do it. We put this section first because you may need to plunge right into ideas that you can put into action immediately.

Section Two is a primer—it includes the things you might want to know about depression, mental health care professionals and potential treatments. This is the more textbook-like section of our handbook, and is designed to be read when you are ready to know more about the details of this illness and the kinds of help available.

Once again, our goal is to help you navigate a difficult time in your life. We hope our handbook will be helpful along your journey. With that in mind, we begin.

a few facts about depression

There is a lot of stigma attached to having an illness like depression—as a society we just don't like to talk about it. We feel guilty and ashamed—about having it, even about having it in our family. But the simple fact is that depression is an illness, just like any other illness you or your child might have, and, just like any other illness, depression should be treated.

EXACTLY WHAT IS DEPRESSION?

First and foremost, depression is a medical term that defines a specific illness. It's more than just a sad or depressed mood, which most of us feel from time to time.

Depression, also called Major Depression or Major Depressive Disorder, is a sustained depressed mood, feeling of sadness, loss of interest or pleasure in most activities, sense of worthlessness and/or guilt, and difficulty with concentration, thinking and making decisions. Some people with depression feel irritable as well.

Frequently, and especially in children and adolescents, these psychological symptoms are accompanied by physical symptoms which can include agitation, fatigue, changes in sleeping patterns, appetite and/or weight, slowed speech and movement, headache, stomach-ache and other aches and pains.

Some depressions are mild and one can function somewhat normally. Some are severe, limiting even the most routine daily activities or leading to thoughts of death or attempts

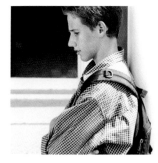 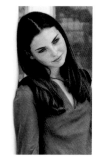

at suicide. Most depressions last for seven to nine months, though some last longer than that.

Those who suffer from an episode of depression are at a higher risk of having other, usually more severe, episodes during their lifetime. *Thus, depression is increasingly being viewed as an illness to be managed with treatment and lifestyle changes, rather than one that will be cured—it's more like diabetes than the flu.*

Roughly two-thirds of children and adolescents with depression have another mental disorder. Dysthymia (see Section Two), anxiety disorders, conduct disorder, substance-related disorders, ADHD (attention deficit-hyperactivity disorder) and learning disorders are the most common co-occurring disorders.

We used to believe that only adults suffered from depression. We now know it can strike anyone, even very young children. Studies tell us that in any given year, as many as 8% of our teenagers and 2.5% of our children are suffering with the illness. *That's too many of our young people suffering,* and, as we noted before, most go undiagnosed and untreated.

There are questions, without definitive answers, about whether and how best to treat depression, particularly in children and adolescents. Although research is ongoing, the studies are not easy to draw firm conclusions from. It's inherently difficult to study mental disorders like depression precisely because the symptoms are primarily psychological rather than physical in nature. In addition, the studies often have flaws—they are short term or conducted in research rather than real-life settings, for example. Finally, and understandably, there are ethical concerns about studying these disorders in children and adolescents.

Our mothers told us to get a good night's sleep, eat healthily and get plenty of exercise—and they were right. These common sense ideas often help reduce the symptoms of depression.

Research is currently being done on the benefits of relaxation techniques such as meditation, breathing exercises and yoga. Incorporating these activities may help as well.

All of this leaves us with a muddy picture of how to best treat depression in our youngsters.

However, despite the inconclusive scientific data, *decades of clinical evidence and a consensus in the mental health community suggest that treatment can help a patient recover from an episode of depression.*

Common sense argues for treatment as well—it just makes sense that treating depression to lessen its length or severity will alleviate pain and suffering and will allow our children to get on with their lives.

We discuss depression in more detail in Section Two, but we wanted at least to set the stage for why you should consider having your child assessed and treated if you think he or she is suffering from depression. And so we move on to just that subject—getting help.

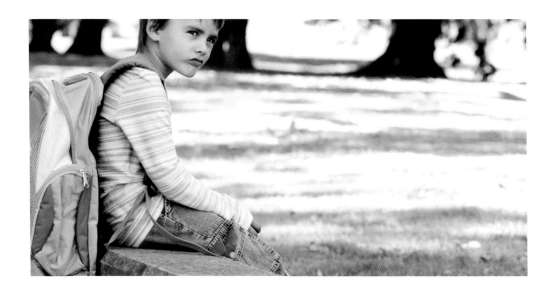

READING OUR HANDBOOK. For ease of reading, we use "he" to refer to your child and "she" to refer to doctors, therapists, teachers, etc. Please indulge us with this convention as you read.

where to begin

It's normal for parents who think their child is suffering from depression to wonder whether they should just wait and see or whether they should seek help.

If you think something is amiss, trust your instinct. If you are unsure, ask a close friend or family member their opinion. The bottom line is, don't hesitate. It's better to err on the side of caution than to wait—and possibly watch your child become increasingly depressed.

Is this an emergency? If your child is in imminent danger of hurting himself or another person, is hearing voices, or is seeing things that aren't there, he may need an immediate evaluation at a hospital.

Either go directly to your hospital or call 9-1-1 for help. Call your child's physician and/or therapist on the way to the hospital to tell them what's going on and get their advice.

Your first phone call should be to your child's physician. Why? Family physicians see thousands of children over their years of practice and are good at determining whether or not there is an issue that needs treatment.

The physician should ask to see your child for a physical examination and to run some tests to make sure that nothing else is wrong; some illnesses, like diabetes, thyroid disease and adrenal gland disease, can act like depression and need to be ruled out.

Before you visit the doctor, take some time to jot down your concerns—moods, behaviors and physical symptoms you are seeing in your child:
- [ ] I think there is a problem because _____ .
- [ ] I heard my child say _____ .
- [ ] I saw my child do _____ .
- [ ] My child is feeling _____ .
- [ ] This is not my child's normal behavior because _____ .
- [ ] I've seen this change in my child over the past ____ weeks or ____ months.

If the doctor agrees with you that there is a problem, she may offer to prescribe medication to see if that helps alleviate the symptoms. While this may seem to be an easy way to proceed, it's best to see a professional—someone who specializes in mental health—to get a formal mental health assessment. Just as the doctor needs to rule out diseases that act like depression, so someone trained in the field of mental health needs to determine exactly what's going on with your child. Proper treatment depends on an accurate diagnosis.

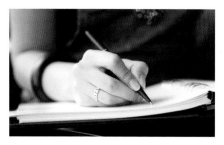

WHAT IS A MENTAL HEALTH ASSESSMENT?

A mental health assessment is one or a series of interviews and tests designed to give you [1] a diagnosis, and [2] a treatment plan.

Often mental health assessments are reasonably simple—one session can be sufficient to give you a working diagnosis and treatment plan. Sometimes a more complete evaluation is needed. If your child's behavior or mood is severe, you may need a formal assessment— a battery of tests—which might include:

[ ] Interviews with and questionnaires for your child, you and other family members

[ ] Interviews with mental health professionals who have worked with your child and/or your family

[ ] Psychological testing of your child's emotional and cognitive functioning

[ ] Neuropsychological testing of your child's thinking and information-processing capabilities

[ ] Psycho-social assessments of your child's interactions with others

[ ] A review of school records, such as report cards

[ ] An evaluation of family dynamics

[ ] A medical evaluation, which could include blood tests and neurological testing of the brain (an EEG and/or MRI).

Keep a journal. Possibly the best piece of advice we can give at the outset is to keep a journal. You can start the journal by including the notes that you took to the doctor, any test results from your visit, behaviors, moods and physical symptoms you are seeing at home or hearing about from school, and changes in your child's relationships with family members and friends.

Try to keep up with it regularly—it will be a great aid to refer to as your child goes through his treatment.

HOW DO YOU FIND SOMEONE TO DO THE ASSESSMENT?

Psychiatrists and psychologists generally have more formal training in assessment than social workers—if your child has a complicated or severe illness, you may want to have the assessment done by one of these two professionals.

Mental health assessments are done by people who specialize in mental health—psychiatrists, psychologists and social workers. The mental health field is generally one of individual practitioners or small groups of professionals working together, so, like finding physicians, most people find someone to do an assessment by asking people they know—friends, neighbors, other parents, school personnel and members of the clergy—for referrals.

Your child's physician is probably the easiest way to find a therapist to do an assessment for your child. She also may be able to help you get an appointment—practices are often booked well in advance and it can be very helpful to have someone open a door for you.

Taking the extra step to get an assessment may seem unnecessary—you may, understandably, want to get your child directly into therapy. But, taking the time up front to get an assessment may pay off in the long run.

If, however, you are waiting for an assessment and your child is getting worse, it might be best to get your child into therapy immediately (see the next section) and come back to the assessment later if the treatment is not working or if you believe the diagnosis you received is not correct.

In addition to getting referrals from your child's physician or people you know, you can call a local mental health social service agency or clinic. Many of these institutions perform assessments, often at reduced rates. The appendix at the back of the handbook has a list of these organizations in the northern suburbs of Chicago.

Whichever source you use, it's important to find someone to do the assessment who has seen a wide variety of cases, who has a broad depth of experience at diagnosing mental disorders, and who has experience working with children who are similar in age to your child.

A FEW THINGS TO NOTE ABOUT ASSESSMENTS

Depression and similar disorders are not always easy to diagnose. It's sometimes difficult to tell which disorder or group of disorders is present, and it can often take several sessions to make a correct diagnosis. As we noted before, many children and adolescents with depression also suffer from another mental disorder.

FOR EASE OF READING, we use the term "therapist" in our handbook to refer to all three mental health professions. In reality, this term and the term "psychotherapist" generally refer to someone who does talk therapy—a psychologist or social worker. A psychiatrist is typically referred to simply as a psychiatrist.

Some disorders can look like depression, but they are not. A good example of this is bipolar disorder. It's very similar to depression until a manic cycle sets in, but it may be several sessions before the manic cycle presents itself to the therapist so that she can accurately identify it.

Diagnosing children is tricky. Children and adolescents—especially children—are often unable to verbalize their feelings—they may not be at a developmental stage that allows them to recognize their feelings and put them into words. Also, children and adolescents are growing rapidly, both physically and mentally. Their moods and behaviors—the manifestations of the disorder—may change along with their growth. Furthermore, some behavior is appropriate at one age, and not another (think temper tantrums)—but children and adolescents can vary greatly from the norm in their developmental stages.

A good diagnostician should consider all of these factors. She should look at whether the symptoms are occurring with unusual frequency, lasting for an abnormal length of time, or occurring at an unexpected time during your child's development. Taking all of these factors into account during the assessment is important because the treatment plan will depend on them.

COMPLETING THE ASSESSMENT

When your child has completed his assessment, it's a good idea to meet with the therapist to discuss the diagnosis and talk about treatment. If there is a report, get a copy of it and read it. It should include both a diagnosis and treatment plan. Write down questions that you have. Here are some to think about:

[ ] How did you arrive at the diagnosis? How certain are you of it?

[ ] Can you tell me about the illness? What are its symptoms? What is its usual course? Where can I get more information about it?

[ ] Can you tell me about the treatment plan you propose? How does it work? Is this the usual treatment plan for this illness (if not, why did you choose it)? What are the benefits? What are the risks? Are there alternatives? How much time is usually involved in treatment? Is it supported by research? Where can I get more information about the treatment plan and the current research on it?

After your meeting, you are ready to continue to the next step—finding the right help for your child.

Involve your child. Ask him to attend the meeting with you. Often, children go through testing, but aren't told what the results of the tests are. If you include your child in the process, he will be better able to understand that it's not "him"— that it's the illness making him feel the way he does. This can be an important step towards him learning to take ownership of and manage his illness.

In the end, if you don't feel comfortable with the diagnosis, or are unsure about the treatment plan, talk to the therapist, (and perhaps your child's physician) about your concerns. Or ask for the records and get a second opinion.

finding the right help

There are three treatment options for depression—talk therapy (psychotherapy), medication or a combination of the two. Different kinds of mental health professionals specialize in these different treatments.

- *Psychiatrists* prescribe and monitor medication. Many psychiatrists only prescribe and monitor medication; they do not practice talk therapy—but some do both.
- *Psychologists and social workers* practice talk therapy, and often specialize in one particular type of therapy. They are not physicians and therefore they cannot prescribe or monitor medication.

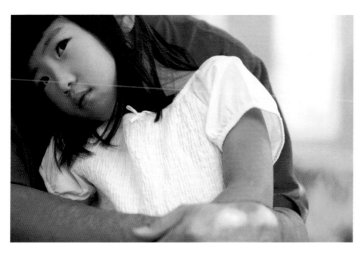

Since different kinds of therapists do different things, it can be confusing to find the right person to help your child. To add to the confusion, the mental health community is fragmented—most therapists have private practices, which sometimes makes finding them difficult.

So, given all of this, how do you find the right person?

We have more information about the different kinds of therapists and therapies in SECTION TWO.

The treatment plan should tell you what kind of therapist your child needs—it's a good starting point to begin to assemble a list of people who may be right for your child.

As with the assessment process, you will probably find your child's therapist through referrals. You can begin by asking your child's physician for her recommendations—and once again perhaps she can make a phone call to open the door for you. The person who did the initial assessment may have some names too—in fact, she may become your child's therapist, certainly a convenient option if the personality fit is right.

Networking in your community is also a good way to find names of therapists, and can be an especially good way to find out which therapists are well regarded, and which are not. **In fact, parents who have been through similar circumstances may be your best sources.**

If your child needs to see more than one therapist—both a psychiatrist to prescribe medication and a talk therapist—finding one may help you find the other. Psychiatrists and talk therapists work regularly with one another and may have a good recommendation for the other half of the team.

Local mental health social service agencies and clinics can be a good source too. The appendix at the back of the handbook will give you a list of these organizations in the northern suburbs of Chicago.

At this point, you may be wondering about treatment. Is it safe? Is it effective? There is a lot of controversy today about these two questions. Mental disorders, by their very nature, are difficult to study and therefore different studies have reached different conclusions over the years.

Most mental health professionals, and the American Psychological Association, in its 2006 *Report of the Working Group on Psychotropic Medications for Children and Adolescents*, recommend a conservative approach for treating children and adolescents who have depression—psychotherapy first, with regular monitoring, followed by carefully controlled medication (usually one of the SSRI antidepressants) together with the psychotherapy if the psychotherapy alone is not effective.

If, however, your child is having significant difficulty with daily functioning, has particularly peculiar thinking or behavior, is focused on death, has attempted suicide, or is engaging in self-injury like cutting, it may be best to begin with medication and psychotherapy together.

If the situation is extremely dire— if your child is an immediate threat to himself or others or if he is hearing voices or seeing things that aren't there, you may need to consider hospitalization.

Although you will see all sorts of therapists listed on the Internet, and many tempting programs, it's unwise to use only the Internet to find a therapist.

A better use of the Internet is to use trusted websites to compile a preliminary list of potential therapists, and then cull that list using personal references you have received from friends, neighbors and professionals in your community.

The Internet can also be of help. Most mental health professional organizations have options on their websites to help you find a therapist in your area. Here are some that may be particularly helpful:

[] The American Psychological Association (*www.apa.org*)
[] The National Association of Social Workers (*www.socialworkers.org*)
[] The American Academy of Child and Adolescent Psychiatry (*www.aacap.org*)
[] Mental Health America (*www.nmha.org*)
[] The Child and Adolescent Bipolar Foundation (*www.bpkids.org*).

Hospital websites may also be helpful, particularly if your child suffers from a particular disorder like an eating disorder.

A list of five to ten names should be sufficient to get you started with the process of finding the right therapist for your child. Why so many? Often therapists are not currently taking new patients (though if you call back in a week or two, their practice may be open)

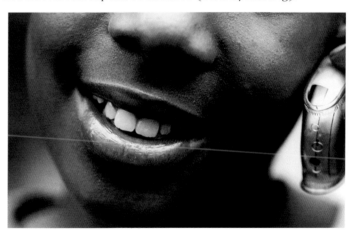

and some therapists, though a good fit for one child, may not be the right person for your child. If a therapist is not taking new patients, ask her for a recommendation.

INTERVIEWING THERAPISTS

Once you have compiled your list, call each person to see whether she is available and willing to treat your child and whether you think she would be a good therapist for your child. You might have to call a few times; many therapists do their own scheduling and are hard to reach. If you think the person is potentially a good fit for your child, set up an interview with her. You will probably want to limit the number of therapists you interview to three or four—this will probably be sufficient for you to find someone who will work well with your child.

At the interview, tell the therapist about your child—age, gender, the reasons (i.e., the moods, behaviors and physical symptoms) that led you to seek help, and the results of your child's mental health assessment. Ask the therapist about her practice and her philosophy towards therapy. Here are some questions you can also ask during the interview:

[ ] How long have you been practicing therapy?
[ ] What kind of therapy do you practice? Is it in line with my child's diagnosis and treatment plan?
[ ] Do you have special training in, or particular experience with, any particular disorder?
[ ] Do you have special training to treat children and/or adolescents?
[ ] Do you work regularly with my child's age group? Gender?
[ ] Do you feel comfortable treating my child, based on his diagnosis, treatment plan, age and gender?
[ ] How often would you see my child?
[ ] Can my child contact you if he needs to talk about an issue in between sessions? How?
[ ] How do you know whether the therapy is working?
[ ] How can my child tell whether the therapy is working?
[ ] Do you set goals with your patients?
[ ] How do you work with families? Do you generally recommend family therapy?
[ ] Will you meet with me regularly to talk about my child's progress? How frequently? How openly can you discuss what goes on in therapy with me?
[ ] How can I contact you to let you know if something is happening at home or school?
[ ] How can I tell whether the therapy is working?
[ ] Have you ever had a patient who was not a good fit, or whose therapy was not working? How did you handle that situation?
[ ] How would you work with other professionals in my child's life— my child's physician, another therapist, school personnel?
[ ] How do you handle emergency situations?
[ ] How do we know when it's time to end therapy?

Involve your child in this final selection process if you think it's appropriate. Children and adolescents, not surprisingly, often resist the idea of therapy. You may get more buy-in from them if you include them.

Your child's relationship with his therapist is a key to successful therapy. The right personality fit is important.

Some children, like some adults, work better with therapists who are more touchy/feely and some work better with therapists who are more pragmatic or business-like in their approach. Take your child's personality into account when you are interviewing therapists and ask yourself, *"Do I think this therapist will be a good fit for my child?"*

If your child has more than one illness—depression and an eating disorder, for example—ask the therapist if she has experience with both conditions.

If your child is young, it's important to find someone who works with your child's age group. The younger the child, the greater the difficulty he will have verbalizing his feelings. Special types of therapy may need to be considered. Play, movement or art therapy, for example, might be particularly useful ways for a young child to express his feelings.

Older children and adolescents are likely to need help with their relationships. Relationships with family members are often troublesome. And friendships, which are particularly important to them and so frequently impaired as a result of depression, may be stressors that are contributing to the depression.

The term "psychotherapist" or "therapist" is not a legal term; rather it's a term we apply broadly to someone who does psychotherapy. Psychiatrists, psychologists and social workers have specific education, training and state licensing in their fields—it's best to make sure your child's therapist is one of these professionals.

In Illinois, you can check to see whether your child's therapist is licensed by going to the Illinois Department of Financial and Professional Regulation's website at *www.idfpr.com* and clicking on "License Look-up Information."

If the therapist—psychiatrist—is going to prescribe medication for your child, ask her about her general philosophy on the use of medication to treat depression in children and adolescents. Some psychiatrists are less committed to talk therapy in addition to medication to treat depression—however, talk therapy **should** be part of the treatment plan.

If the therapist—psychiatrist—is going to prescribe medication for your child, make sure you ask how often and which tests or assessments she will use to assess both the effectiveness and side effects of the medication. Of course, it goes without saying that frequent and in-depth monitoring is very important. Some of these medications require regular blood tests to monitor toxicity.

Once you have selected your child's therapist, it's time to begin therapy.

getting treatment

It's not always easy to get your child to go to therapy. We all want to feel that we're normal and there is a considerable amount of stigma in our society about therapy. Don't be surprised if your child thinks he doesn't need therapy, or if he resists going. Explain to your child that going to therapy is not a punishment; it's a chance for him get through a difficult time and to learn coping strategies that he will use for the rest of his life. Try to keep an upbeat, but firm, stance on the issue.

Your child might be fearful or anxious about going to therapy. This, too, is normal. Acknowledging that you know it's a scary thing for your child might be just what he needs to help him overcome that initial, and understandable, fear.

Often the biggest barrier to getting your child to go to therapy is denial—it's normal for children, and adults, to deny there is a problem, or deny that they need treatment to help solve the problem.

Watch for moments of opportunity to tap into—moments when your child is vulnerable, when your child knows he needs help, and may be willing to reach out for it. Even if your child is in some degree of self-denial about his illness, such moments exist and they can be breakthrough moments.

"YOU DESERVE TO FEEL BETTER"

If your child is tearful day after day or is withdrawing from activities he previously enjoyed, you may be able to gently broach the subject of therapy. Sometimes just saying, "You deserve to feel better," can open the door to getting him the help he needs.

Keep in mind, too, that therapists are very familiar with the problem of patients who don't want to go to therapy. If you can persuade your child to make two or three visits, that may be enough for the therapist to make a good connection with him. You should be able to tell if it's working—if your child begins to go to therapy sessions more and more willingly, that's a good sign.

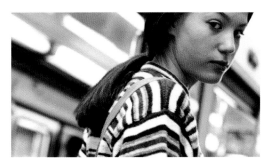

Adolescents, in particular, may balk at therapy. They often feel that by right they should be able to determine their own course of action. To a certain extent, that is true.

One thing is clear—you can't make someone do something they don't want to do. You can only present the options for them, and tell them why you think it's a good idea to go. *Successful therapy requires that the person in therapy eventually take ownership of his own mental health—and that goes for our children as well as us.* But often, gentle, but firm, prodding can go a long way towards getting a reluctant child or adolescent to go to therapy.

STARTING THERAPY

Once you have cleared the initial hurdle of going to therapy, it's time to turn your attention to the therapy itself. You, your child and his therapist should have an initial "getting started" meeting. If you didn't do so during the preliminary interview, give the therapist a general history of your child—moods and behavior patterns, a health history, and school performance information.

You should also tell the therapist about your child's past health history—other mental disorders, ADHD or learning disorders, allergies, other chronic illnesses and medications, including over-the-counter medications, vitamins and herbal supplements, that your child is taking.

If your child has a history of using tobacco, alcohol or street drugs, the therapist should know that as well.

Think about it as telling your child's story—the more you can paint a picture of your child, his likes and dislikes, his skills and his temperament, the more the therapist will begin to understand your child. Bring your journal to the meeting.

Your child can tell his story from his perspective.

Ask your child's talk therapist about therapy and what to expect from it.
- [ ] What do the diagnosis and treatment plan mean?
- [ ] What happens during therapy sessions?
- [ ] How frequently will sessions take place?
- [ ] What changes in mood, behavior and physical symptoms will you look for? How soon do you expect them to occur?
- [ ] What changes will my child feel or notice?
- [ ] What changes will we see at home?

[ ] How can the family help?

[ ] Are family therapy sessions needed?

[ ] What can the school do to help?

[ ] Will there be "therapy homework?"

[ ] How frequently should we meet to talk about progress?

[ ] How can I contact you to let you know about important issues at home and school?

[ ] How will you work with my child's physician, other therapist and school personnel?

[ ] How can we reach you during an emergency?

[ ] What should we do if a session is missed without excuse?

[ ] How do you know when therapy isn't working? What do you do in those situations?

[ ] How do you know when therapy should be ended?

If your child is going to begin medication as part of his treatment, ask the psychiatrist about the medication she is proposing for your child:

[ ] How does the medication work?

[ ] Which symptoms will the medication alleviate? How long will it be before we see positive results? Do the symptoms disappear all at once or gradually over time?

[ ] How do you know when the medication is working?

[ ] What are the side effects of the medication? What should we do if they occur? Which are serious and which are not? What should we do in the case of a sudden negative side effect?

[ ] How long do you think my child will be on this medication?

[ ] How often will you see my child to monitor the medication?

[ ] What kind of tests will you run to make sure the medication is safe for my child? How often will you do these tests?

[ ] How should the medication be taken? Regularly, at a certain time of day? With or without food, liquids or other medications? Are there any foods or other substances that should be avoided?

[ ] What should we do if a dose is missed?

[ ] What are the potential interactions with other medications, over-the-counter products, tobacco, alcohol, and street drugs?

[ ] Where can I get more information about this medication? Is it approved for use for my child's illness? My child's age group? Can I see the research on the medication?

[ ] What are the long term risks of the medication?

For more information about medication used to treat depression, see SECTION TWO, Chapter Four.

A FEW IDEAS

If your child is taking medication, it's a good idea to keep a medication journal.
Psychotropic medication takes a while to get right and is frequently adjusted, both the
dose and the type—keeping a regular record is a valuable tool to
use to determine whether adjustments are needed. Use it to record
every time your child takes his medication, the dose taken, and daily
reports of feelings, moods, behaviors, physical symptoms, benefits and side effects of the
medication. You and your child can both participate in the maintenance of this journal.

Psychotropic: aimed specifically
at treating mental disorders.

**If your child is taking medication, you should make sure that both of his therapists
speak to one another regularly.** And, make sure your child knows that he can't stop the
talk therapy just because he is on medication. Both are
important steps towards your child's recovery.

Ask your child's therapist about goal-setting—it's
a tool some therapists use. Goal-setting is a process in
which the therapist and your child set specific, tangible
goals and measurements, or signposts, which they use
to assess the progress that's being made in therapy.

For example, one goal they might set is a decrease in
your child's depressive feelings. The measurements for
that goal might be that your child smiles more often at
home and joins an extracurricular activity after school.

Or they might set a goal of better sleep patterns,
and the signposts might be that your child is able
to maintain a regular bedtime schedule and wakes
feeling refreshed each morning.

The benefit of goal-setting is that it provides a steady
and regular tool to help assess whether therapy is
proceeding well or not. If the goals are not met,
therapy can be adjusted.

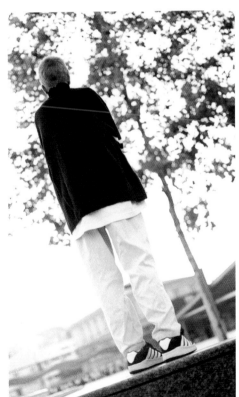

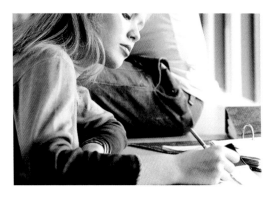

Another tool some therapists use is a journal— "therapy homework" for your child. Journals can take many forms and be tailored to your child's skills and needs—it can be the traditional kind of journal in which your child writes about his thoughts, moods and feelings, but it can also be something as simple as an art journal—drawings done by your child—or a sticker journal, in which your child places stickers to record his moods.

Don't forget about your journal too. Your continuing observations about your child's moods, behaviors and physical symptoms are important.

ONE MORE THING

There is one more thing you should think about with respect to your child's therapy. In order for your child's therapy to be successful, you and members of your family may need to participate in family therapy. While this can seem like one more thing on your plate, it can be a very useful thing for the child who is suffering from depression, not to mention the family as a whole—sometimes depression is part of a family dynamic and sometimes one member's depression can create a negative family dynamic.

Ask your child's therapist if she thinks your child would benefit from family therapy. She can probably help you find a family therapist.

MONITORING THERAPY

Once your child (and perhaps the entire family) is established in therapy, goals are set and journals are being kept, you've made a lot of progress. You should feel good about that. But ... you're not done. At some point, say a month or so into therapy, and then from time to time during the course of your child's therapy, you should check in with your child and meet with your child's therapist to assess whether therapy is going well and whether your child's therapist is a good fit.

These are sometimes tricky questions to ask and there are not always easy answers to them. Therapy is between your child and his therapist. Furthermore, even asking the question begs the next question—what to do if it's not going well. However, these questions need to be asked; you don't want to waste precious time if the therapist isn't a good fit, or if the therapy isn't working.

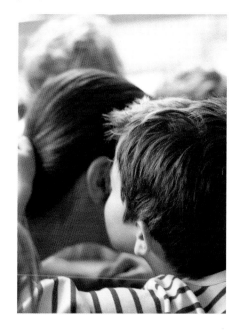

One way to get a sense of how therapy is going is to sit down with your child and ask him what he thinks.

[ ] How do you feel compared to before you began therapy?
[ ] Do you like your therapist?
[ ] Do you feel respected and comfortable talking to your therapist?
[ ] Do you think she is helping you?
[ ] Do you think you are progressing on your goals?

Depending on your child's age and temperament, you may want to ask to take a look at his journal if he's keeping one. But be sensitive about this issue—an older child may feel you are prying if you ask this.

Keep in mind a few things when you talk to your child about therapy. The younger the child, the less he may be able to talk about therapy. And, of course, if your child is going to therapy under protest, he may not be the best judge of the effectiveness of the therapy. If your child responds that he hates therapy or it's "stupid" or "pointless," that may not necessarily be the objective case—in fact, it may be difficult for him precisely **because** it's working.

If your child is on medication, ask your child whether he thinks the medication is working, and if he notices any benefits or any negative side effects. The medication journal will be a good reference point to use here. Make sure you report any side effects to your child's psychiatrist so she can make adjustments to the medication if need be.

In addition to asking your child about therapy, you should meet with your child's therapist and ask her what her impressions are:

[ ] Do you agree with the initial diagnosis?

[ ] Tell me about your relationship with my child. Do you think you work well together?

[ ] Are you making satisfactory progress towards meeting your goals? Can we review the goals and the progress that's being made?

[ ] How much more time do you think you will need for treatment?

[ ] Are there things we should be doing at home to help?

[ ] Are there things that the school, other therapist or other professionals should be doing?

[ ] Are family sessions recommended?

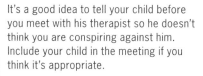

It's a good idea to tell your child before you meet with his therapist so he doesn't think you are conspiring against him. Include your child in the meeting if you think it's appropriate.

If your child is seeing both a psychiatrist and a talk therapist, ask both therapists how often and effectively they are speaking to one another to coordinate treatment.

Keep in mind when talking to both your child and his therapist(s) that they may be unwilling, or unable, to speak about the details of therapy. Confidentiality is an important part of therapy. Your child needs to know that his therapist will not tell you everything that they are working on in therapy—it needs to be a safe environment for your child to talk about his feelings, which may include feelings about you. On the other hand, the therapist should be forthcoming with you about the success or failure of the therapy, goals, timelines and other more general topics.

A word of caution. Be a little careful about setting up a dynamic where you are calling or meeting with your child's therapist too frequently for a status check. It can be seen by your child, especially if he is older, as interfering. It can also offer your child a handy excuse to avoid taking ownership of his therapy—*if mom or dad is overseeing it, then I don't have to.* Keep in mind that therapy is your child's job, not yours.

If your child is on medication, be sure to bring the medication journal along when you meet with the psychiatrist. Talk about both the benefits and negative side effects of the medication. Ask how much longer the psychiatrist believes your child will be on the medication. Also ask how she is assessing the effectiveness, and how is she measuring the side effects and safety of the medication.

If you and your child believe the medication is not working as effectively as it should or if the side effects are a nagging problem, talk to the psychiatrist about changing medications or adjusting the dose. It can often take a while to get the medication right and you, your child and his psychiatrist may need to be persistent in that effort.

Sometimes you can tell whether your child is progressing in therapy by looking at their writing or art at school. If there are projects at school that might give you an insight into his emotional state, ask his teacher if you can see his work.

Again, you need to tread carefully here, especially with older children and adolescents. Looking at their private writing without their permission might provoke their ire, at a price that isn't worth what you got from it.

You also are a good touchstone as to whether you think therapy is working well. Review your journal and ask yourself these questions:

[ ] Do I see improvement in my child's mood, behavior and/or physical symptoms?
[ ] Is my child meeting his goals?
[ ] Does my child like his therapist?
[ ] Is the therapist communicating openly and regularly with me?
[ ] Is the therapist accessible to my child?
[ ] Do I think the therapist is helping my child?
[ ] Do I think the therapist is a good fit for my child?

If, after talking to your child and sitting down with his therapist, you are concerned about the progress, or are worried that the fit isn't right between the therapist and your child, talk to the therapist about your concerns. It can be tempting to make a change to another therapist

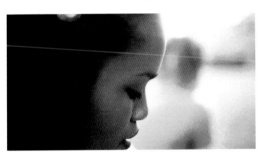

and it's often done and often necessary—but it isn't always a good idea. You may not be seeing significant progress, but this isn't necessarily a sign that therapy isn't working—it may just mean that the hard, sometimes unpleasant, work of therapy is occurring and the benefits are yet to come. "Shopping around" for different therapists when issues get tough, complex or challenging is not helpful to your child.

If, however, in the end, you come to the conclusion that you need to make a change, do so. The relationship between therapist and patient is critical to the success of the therapy, and if you conclude that the relationship just isn't there, or you are unhappy at the progress being made after having given it fair time, it's probably best to begin the process all over again and find another therapist.

This is often easier said than done—it took a lot of effort to find a therapist in the first place, and it is even more difficult to come to the conclusion that the therapist you worked so hard to find just isn't working out. In addition, your child may not want to make a change, or he may take the opportunity to lobby hard for discontinuation of therapy altogether, for the very understandable reason that he has to start all over again. If you find yourself at this place, the list you compiled at the beginning of the process will be a help to you as you travel down this path again.

WORKING TOGETHER

When your child is suffering from depression, one of your jobs is to make sure that the other adults who are a part of your child's daily life—teachers, coaches, tutors, etc.—are aware of what's going on to the extent they need to be. Why? If the right people know about your child's illness—not necessarily the details, but at least the gist—then they can provide a support system for him at times during the day when you are not there. These people can also let you know when they see something that is particularly troublesome, and you can then let your child's therapist know about the concerns.

Also, by keeping in contact with these people, you are in a better position to help your child deal with troublesome events in his life. For example, if your child is having a difficult time at lunchtime with his friends, talking to your child's therapist and the school about the problem may result in some creative strategies; perhaps the school can ask the lunchroom monitor to temporarily "arrange" seating at lunch. Your child and his therapist can then brainstorm strategies that he can use to make lunchtime less difficult to negotiate. Similarly, if your child's teacher or tutor notices a rapid decline in your child's ability to pay attention, she can let you know and you can report this information to your child's therapist.

However, you will want to take your child's privacy into consideration before speaking to these people. As much as we don't like it, stigma is still an issue when it comes to mental disorders, and your goal in taking these people into your family confidence is to provide a safety net for your child, not to embarrass or humiliate him in any way. Perhaps getting permission from your child beforehand will help you decide which adults to speak to and what to say.

You now have your child's therapy firmly in hand, and so now we turn to the home— dealing with your child, other family members … and yourself.

Because school is such an important part of your child's day, we have devoted Chapter Four of SECTION ONE to help you with this subject.

talking to your child

One thing you can do for your child is to let him know that you support him throughout this process. He needs to know that you love him, that you are able to separate out the illness from the "real" person, and that you will always be there when needed.

Talking to your child about his depression is often a tricky, and ever-changing, task. Being honest and open with your child about his condition and treatment is a good place to begin.

As we have said before, your child, like everyone, wants to be "normal," and may deny he has depression. In fact, this is very common. If you keep an open dialogue with your child, over time he may begin to admit that there is a problem and talk to you about it. Reassure him that you know he is in pain—a pain he deserves to be free from.

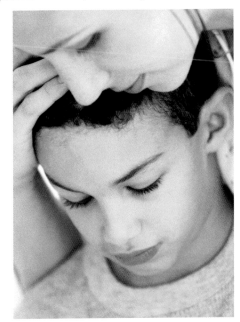

Don't avoid the issue—it's the elephant in the room anyway. Talking can bring you together in ways that will surprise you. But also be prepared for your child to be honest with you about his feelings about you, often unflinchingly, and sometimes dead right. Don't take it too personally and listen, really listen, to what your child is telling you. This may be an important part of his therapy, and it's certainly good modeling for him. Someone in the throes of depression is often touchy about others' criticisms and if you can show him that you can take his constructive criticisms of you, he may begin to do the same.

Talking openly to your child might also foster an atmosphere in which your child can talk to you about other problems he might be having—ancillary problems, like problems with friends or academic issues. Often when a child is depressed, friendships become difficult. Some friends, even long-time ones, may distance themselves from your child.

Your child may be teased by his friends or classmates about his depression. This can be extremely hurtful. If it occurs, let your child's therapist know about it.

Talk to your child about it and let him know that you understand how hurtful this is. Remind him that teasing is often a result of fear. You can brainstorm possible solutions with your child—he can just ignore the teasing or talk to the offender about it, for example.

Be honest with your child. Tell your child that you don't know what the answer to the illness is and that you don't know how or when it will all play out. This is the unhappy truth of dealing with mental disorders—they are unpredictable. But making sure that your child knows that together you will deal with whatever the future holds can be immensely reassuring for him. And of course, tell him that while you may not know the details of how his depression will affect him or when he will get better, make sure you tell him that he **will get better,** with treatment, time—and love.

Your child may separate himself from his friends. It's common for someone who is depressed to have a low level of self-worth. Your child may believe that his friends don't like him. Remind your child that this is the depression speaking—and that he may be perceiving things differently than they really are.

If your child comes to you, or if you see that friendships are changing, you might want to talk to your child about how he can make things better—even just one loyal friend can be a significant thing for your child. You should also convey this changing environment to your child's therapist so that she can deal with the issue during therapy.

Your child's relationship with his siblings may also suffer. Siblings often don't understand what is happening, and may be embarrassed, angry, scared or jealous. To make matters more complicated, irritability is a common symptom of depression and siblings are sometimes a target for a depressed child who needs to let off steam (and vice-versa). It can be a tricky situation for you to mediate—but open communication with everyone in the family may help diffuse some of the tension. And family therapy may be an immeasurably useful tool to help everyone in the family deal with these natural tensions.

Another change that you may see is a decline in your child's interest in schoolwork and other activities. A depressed child feels hopeless and may also be struggling with fatigue—he is likely not too interested in doing homework—or even playing in the back yard after school. You may find yourself spending quite a bit of time monitoring these activities—checking in from time to time with teachers, coaches, etc., and trouble-shooting problems. You may need to be an advocate for your child, especially when times are particularly difficult.

Some children need a break from activities when they are suffering from depression—it may be just too difficult to keep up with schoolwork *and* baseball *and* piano lessons. On the other hand, if your child can stick with some activities that he used to find pleasure in, even just one activity, it may become a valuable part of your child's recovery. Like everything else, it's a balancing act.

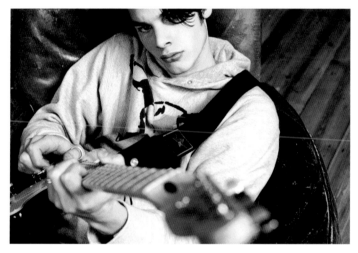

But—you will have to choose your battles and, remember, you don't want to win the battle to lose the war. Some activities may need to be dropped and sometimes you need to insist on follow through … and follow through yourself to make sure your child keeps up with his responsibilities. The more responsibility your child can take for his daily functions, the better. Encourage this and praise it when it occurs.

Your child may need special adjustments at school to help him manage the school day, at least for a while. We have more information on the kinds of help available at school in Chapter Four.

Again, please remember that it will be helpful for your child's recovery if you share all of these at-home issues with your child's therapist so that they can be dealt with in therapy as well as at home.

talking to your family

As if dealing with your suffering child is not enough, you will quickly discover that what your child is feeling has repercussions in your family—both immediate and extended. The child who is suffering may have feelings and questions about his place in the family. Siblings, you, your spouse, extended family—all have different feelings, reactions—and opinions—about what is going on.

**If your child is dealing with depression,
the whole family is dealing with depression.**

Family members will have a myriad of feelings and questions about the condition and behavior of your child. They may be embarrassed, anxious, angry, afraid. They may communicate this to you—they may not.

Siblings can be especially impacted by the illness of another child in the family. And each sibling, of course, will react in her own way. It is common for siblings to be embarrassed about what's going on—the stigma associated with depression is significant.

Siblings are also often angry or jealous; they are not getting the attention they are used to. And they may be afraid, wondering if they are the next one in the family to "get" depression. If you explain to them what's going on, and help them address their feelings or vent to you about their worry or frustrations, you may be able to help them move to a more positive stance, become more sensitive to the suffering and pain of depression, and even to help support their suffering sibling.

It's important to respect your child's right to his privacy about his depression.

Talking to your child before speaking to other family members will help give you an idea what information your child feels comfortable sharing with other family members, and what information he would prefer to keep private.

To the extent you are honest and reassuring with all the members of your family about what's going on, you will serve the entire family well—they will see your modeling and may begin to adopt it themselves. If you treat this as an illness, just like any other illness—which it is—and not a black mark on your child or a permanent personality trait, the rest of the family hopefully will begin to treat it in a similar manner.

But know that this is a process, not a one-time conversation. Remember that your child's siblings are children themselves—all the intellectual conversation in the world may not help them understand that it's the depression talking and not their brother the next time he shouts at them for no good reason or once again gets a bye from you on dishwashing duty.

Try to maintain normal family activities. Go to the movies together. Plan an outing. Eating together even a few nights a week can be an important way of keeping the family together.

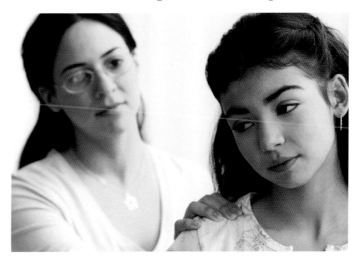

Don't forget family therapy—it may help you resolve some of the family dynamic issues so that the whole family can find a way to work together in positive ways to support one another.

You may find that certain family members need to seek individual therapy to help them deal with what's going on. This can be very helpful to a family member who may or may not even know what to think, much less how to feel, about this illness that has invaded her life—and it is powerful indeed for the child who is suffering to see that other family members are getting the help they need too.

THREE
at home

taking care of yourself

At this point, you are probably thinking, *Phew! I need support!*

You probably do—you may need to see a therapist yourself. We have found this to be immensely helpful. A therapist can help in several ways. She can help you deal with your own emotions about what's happening. And she is someone you can bounce ideas off of. Finally, and very importantly, getting yourself into therapy is setting a good example for your child.

**You can't be available to the rest of the family
if you don't take care of yourself.**

One emotion you may be feeling is guilt. Parents often are racked by it—they believe they caused the illness, and they feel totally responsible for it. You may even feel family members or friends judging you. Try to deal with this emotion openly with your therapist.

And know that you are not the cause of your child's depression. **You are not the cause.** Understanding this, really believing it, will be a big help to both you and your family.

Another issue that sometimes occurs when a child is suffering from depression is spousal relationships. Sometimes spouses blame one another for the illness, sometimes one spouse doesn't believe there is a problem, sometimes spouses disagree over what to do about the illness. All of these things are pretty common occurrences. We don't have an easy answer to these issues. Just try to remind one another that it's an illness—and try to talk through your disagreements with an open heart and an open mind. Remember, your spouse knows your child as well as you do and may have a perspective you've never even considered—and he may even be right!

Try to agree, or at least agree to disagree, on the steps you are taking and, remember too that this is a journey and no one decision will make or break your child's recovery. By working together and supporting your child, and his siblings, you will go a long way to stabilizing the family and helping everyone during a difficult time.

You and your spouse may find it beneficial to join a support group. Much like seeing a therapist, talking to people who are in the same place as you are can help in two ways—they can help you deal with your emotions in a safe and understanding environment and they can help you problem-solve some of the daily issues that are difficult for you to sort through.

These organizations can help you find a support group in your area:
[ ] The National Alliance on Mental Illness (*www.nami.org*)
[ ] The Depression and Bipolar Support Alliance (*www.dbsalliance.org*)
[ ] The Child and Adolescent Bipolar Foundation (*www.bpkids.org*).

In addition, many of the organizations listed at the back of the handbook have on-line chat or "ask a professional" resources on their websites.

THREE
at home

You may be hesitant to talk to others about what's going on, but once you begin letting others in, you may be surprised at how many people have been in a similar situation.

Remember the statistics at the beginning of the book. **You are not alone.**

Don't forget your friends. Or your close family members. You should not feel as if you are going through this alone. Call on people close to you to help you—even if it's making dinner for the family or going for a walk. Talking to a trusted friend may be the best thing you do—it's a wonderful thing to be able to confide your darkest fears and deepest emotions to someone who loves you.

And, please, give yourself a little room for errors. You won't be a perfect parent. No one is, even during the best of times. You will make mistakes, both with your child and with the rest of the family. As we ourselves tell our children—recognize when you have made an error, apologize to the people involved and move forward—so you get on with the things that need attending to.

Hopefully, you can also find time to exercise, sleep, eat a healthy diet, and go to a movie or do some other favorite fun thing—these can be stress-relieving activities for you and it's important that you take the time to do them. Remember, you can't be available to the rest of family if you don't take care of yourself.

one final thought

Therapy is a journey.

Recovery won't happen overnight. It will take time—you will have setbacks. Expect this at the outset, and know that if you keep at it, even through the setbacks, you will eventually reap the rewards of your hard work—a recovered child, able to get on with life and having learned an important life lesson—that everyone is confronted with difficult issues during the course of their lives, but that resiliency and hard work can be the key to managing through those difficult times.

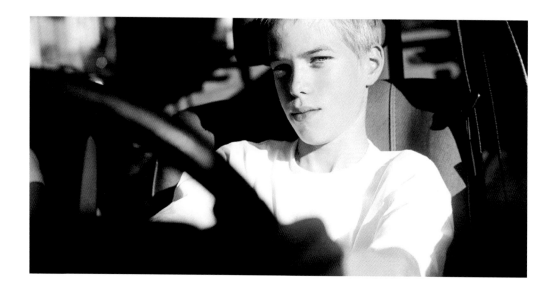

talking to the school

It's common for parents to hesitate telling anyone at school what's going on when their child is suffering from depression or any mental disorder. As parents, we want to protect our children. We worry that if we tell someone at school, our child may be treated differently—or looked down upon.

But if you can judiciously talk to school personnel about your child's condition and his needs, you and the school can work together to help your child make the best out of a very important part of his day. You need to make sure the school is a good environment and that it's providing the right services to your child.

Who at the school should know about your child's illness? At the very least, your child's advisor, primary teacher and/or classroom teacher should know what's going on. You should also consider telling your child's favorite teacher—having one adult that your child trusts and can go to during the school day can be an incredibly important safety net.

A few words about medication and school policy. State law stipulates that if your child is on medication with side effects that could occur during the school day, the school must know about it.

If your child needs to take his medication during the school day, the school nurse or a designate must administer it.

Think about contacting the school nurse—she may already have an inkling that there is an issue anyway. Many childhood depressions have physical components to them, like headache or stomach-ache. If the nurse knows ahead of time what's going on with your child, she is in a better position to help if and when your child comes to her office.

It's also important to talk to one or more of the school's mental health staff—psychologist, social worker or counselor. These people can help your child with his school-related issues. They may also be able to help your child's teacher understand how to make the classroom experience better for your child.

How and what should you tell the school? The way we most effectively communicate with others is face-to-face, so we suggest you begin there. Ask for a meeting with those people you think should know about your child's illness. Consider asking the principal to attend the meeting, particularly if your child is very young, or suffering particularly acutely.

Make sure the school knows the appropriate facts about your child's illness, treatment he is receiving, your thoughts on the ramifications of the illness for your child's progress at school and your ideas about any changes or adjustments your child may need at school.

Who are these people? The school psychologist performs assessments and evaluations for children who may need special adjustments to their school day, a topic which is discussed in detail later in this chapter. She also often conducts counseling sessions at school.

Social workers and counselors have many different functions in the school. They sometimes lead counseling sessions at school. They also are often in classrooms, working with teachers on classroom dynamics, and in the cafeteria or on the playground to observe and be available to students. Social workers also help school psychologists with assessments and evaluations.

You may also want to share information about any social challenges your child is facing. Who your child is sitting with at lunch and whether or not he has been abandoned by friends are important issues. The school should be sensitive to these problems and their effect on your child's ability to function at school.

Think about giving school personnel permission to speak directly with your child's therapist. You can even ask her to attend the meeting. Most therapists are comfortable working with school personnel. But be sure that you talk to her beforehand about which issues she should, and should not, discuss with the school.

It's a good idea to follow up after the meeting with a letter or an email to make sure everyone is on the same page as to the specifics of the discussion, especially if you have come to any agreements with the school about changes to the school day to help your child.

getting help from the school

Now that you've had initial contact with the school, you will want to consider the resources the school has available for your child. We mentioned before that school psychologists or social workers conduct counseling sessions at school. The goal of these sessions is to focus on issues that affect the learning process or other aspects of your child's school day—they may be a real help to your child.

> The goal of counseling sessions at school is to focus on issues that affect your child's learning and functioning at school. It is different from individual therapy done outside the school and shouldn't be seen as an alternative to it.

Group counseling sessions are another option to consider. These sessions are usually organized around a specific topic such as bereavement or divorce, or issues like cutting or eating disorders. Schools often call group therapy sessions by different names—friendship groups, support groups, or social skills groups are all common names. Depending on your child's illness, one of these groups may be helpful to him.

In addition to counseling sessions at school, if your child is having trouble with the school day in a way that significantly affects his ability to learn or to function at school, you may want to, or the school may want you to, consider adjustments to the school day—commonly referred to in educational jargon as modifications, accommodations or interventions—to help your child.

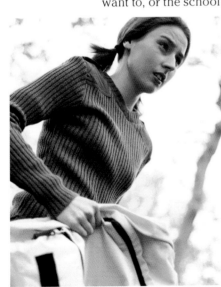

What, exactly, are these adjustments? In general, they are changes to the school day to help your child overcome the disability that's preventing him from being successful at school. They run the gamut from simple changes to very significant and formal ones.

For example, if your child is tired at school because he isn't sleeping well, a simple change like sitting in the front of the class might help him be more attentive in class. On the other end of the spectrum are the more substantive changes—if your child finds the activity of a regular classroom too overwhelming to allow him to concentrate, he might benefit from taking his classes for all or part of the day in a special education classroom with a small group of students, or even one-on-one with a special education teacher.

How can you avail yourself of these adjustments? Well, the simple changes are fairly easily done. They are "informal" agreements that you and the school make together. Very simply, you meet and decide what changes should be made. You can begin this process by requesting a meeting with your child's teacher, school principal and other key staff members. If you come to one of these informal agreements, it's wise to document it in writing. Make sure that everyone, particularly the classroom teacher, has a copy of the agreement so that they can make sure they are following it correctly.

Because these informal adjustments can be implemented immediately, you may want to begin with them if you think your child needs adjustments to his school day. If you can come to an agreement with the school in this manner, it is by far the most expedient way to go, and often offers sufficient changes to the school day to help your child.

The next type of adjustment can be used if your child's illness limits his ability to learn or engage in other activities at school in a more significant way. But they are still relatively simple changes to the school day—like extended testing time.

These adjustments are governed by a federal law, known as Section 504 of The Rehabilitation Act of 1973, or simply Section 504, and are generally referred to as "modifications" and/or "accommodations." As you might expect with any law, Section 504 sets forth specific requirements that must be met—your child must "[1] have a physical or mental impairment that substantially limits one or more major life activities; [2] have a record of such impairment; or [3] be regarded as having such impairment" to qualify for Section 504.

Some common informal adjustments you may want to consider are:
- Reduced homework expectations.
- Schedule changes, such as taking harder classes later in the day.
- Sitting in the front of the class to improve attentiveness and concentration.
- Advance notice to the teacher that it's a bad day, so that she can be on the watch in case the situation deteriorates.
- An agreed-upon safe place, such as the nurse's office, for your child to go to when he is feeling out of control—and standing permission for him to excuse himself from class when necessary to go to this place.

It's important to regularly monitor informal and Section 504 adjustments to your child's school day—they are not formally overseen at school and busy school staff can sometimes overlook them. Often even little adjustments, if scrupulously followed, can make a big difference in your child's day.

The third and final type of adjustment is the most substantive and formal—and it has the benefit of being monitored on a regular basis by special education staff at the school. These adjustments are called "interventions" and are governed by the federal Individual with Disabilities Education Act, IDEA (which has been updated and is now sometimes referred to by the acronym IDEIA). IDEA/IDEIA interventions are available to students who have a disability that falls into one of thirteen specific categories—serious emotional disturbance is the category that children with mental disorders, including depression, may fall into. The disability must also:

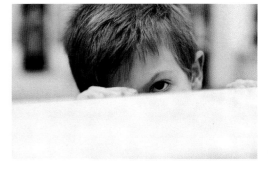

FOUR
at school

Private schools are not required to provide the services required by either Section 504 or IDEA/IDEIA. If your child is at a private school, you will need to work with the school staff to implement informal adjustments.

- adversely affect educational performance, and
- require special education services—a modified curriculum and/or instructional support from special education staff.

THERE'S A NEW GUY IN TOWN.
Congress recently enacted a new law, called Response to Intervention (RtI) that is now being implemented in school districts. RtI is an attempt to cut through the formal process and paperwork of Section 504 and IDEA/IDEIA so that students can receive services more quickly and efficiently. Currently, RtI is being implemented to help students in academic areas, but it will eventually be expanded to cover other areas of impairment. You may want to ask your school whether RtI is an appropriate mechanism under which your child can receive services.

Section 504 and IDEA/IDEIA sound a lot alike. So what's the difference and what's the practical implication of one versus the other? Very simply, IDEA/IDEIA interventions are more substantive changes than the ones available either informally or under Section 504. And they are managed by special education staff. This means that, unlike either informal or Section 504 adjustments, IDEA/IDEIA interventions are overseen on a daily basis by someone at the school to make sure they are being implemented.

However, the downside of both Section 504 and IDEA/IDEIA is that, unlike informal adjustments, you must go through a formal process to obtain services. This can take some time to do.

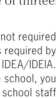

THE PROCESS

The first step in the process of getting help either through Section 504 or IDEA/IDEIA is requesting a "referral." This is a request for an "evaluation" to see whether or not your child is eligible for special services. The school then decides whether or not to proceed with the evaluation. They will do so if they believe that the illness has an "adverse educational effect" on the child. (Remember, this can include non-academic disabilities like depression if they affect the child's ability to learn or function at school.)

What is an evaluation? An evaluation is a variety of tests and a review of your child's performance at school. Depending on his disability or illness, the evaluation may include psychological, cognitive and academic testing, speech, vision and hearing assessments, assessments of the child's learning environment and learning style, reviews of student records, observation of the child in class, behavior rating scales, interviews with parents, and social and health histories of the child.

LEGAL NOTES: Put your request for a referral and evaluation in writing.

When the school agrees to an evaluation and the parent signs a consent for it, the school has 60 school days to complete the evaluation and hold the eligibility meeting.

Evaluations are done by a team of school personnel, typically including the school psychologist, and are done free of charge to the family. If your child has had testing done outside the school—either for his illness or for a learning disability—give this information to the school so they can consider it during the evaluation.

Be sure to document what's taking place and keep copies of all correspondence between you and the school.

If you wish to, you can have an evaluation performed by a professional outside of the school at your own expense. The school is obligated to review the evaluation but it does not have to agree with its conclusions and it may decide to conduct an evaluation of its own.

After the evaluation has taken place, a "multi-disciplinary conference" (MDC), which includes parents and school personnel, takes place. An MDC is an "eligibility meeting" to discuss the child's eligibility for services and for which type of services.

If the school agrees that services are needed, an educational plan will be developed. If services are to be provided under IDEA/IDEIA, an "IEP" (Individualized Educational Plan) will be written that documents the goals and the instructional services and/or modifications to the curriculum to be provided. If services are to be provided under Section 504, a 504 Plan will be written. Make sure you get a copy of whatever plan is developed and read it to be sure it reflects what was agreed upon at the eligibility meeting, or any other

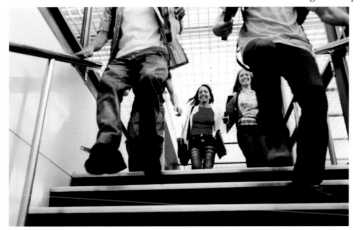

meeting, that you attended. You will be asked to sign these documents—if you are unsure about them, tell the school that you would like more time to consider them (and perhaps consult with your child's therapist or others).

Any services agreed to by the school are free of charge to the parent. If the school is not able to provide them, they are obligated to pay for them.

Both Section 504 and IDEA/IDEIA require that children be put in the most regular or mainstream setting possible. Section 504 requires a student be educated with their non-disabled peers to the extent possible and IDEA/IDEIA requires a child be accommodated in the "least restrictive environment," or LRE.

A FINAL WORD

The issues of adjustments to your child's school day are sometimes difficult—as we said before, mental disorders are often hard to diagnose and difficult for some people to accept as real, so it's probably no surprise that people will differ over whether and how to offer adjustments to the school day to accommodate a mental disorder like depression. Because of this, you may find yourself disagreeing with the school over the issue. If you do, both Section 504 and IDEA/IDEIA provide for an impartial hearing process, called a "due process hearing." You can ask for a hearing at any point in the process. Mediation is one possible way of handling the dispute, and attorneys who specialize in special education law can help you with both mediation and a due process hearing.

FOUR
at school

privacy and school records

What about your child's privacy? When you tell any member of the school community about your child's condition, you can also tell that person who else she may share this information with and who she should not. But keep in mind that this can be a double-edged sword. Your goal is to make sure that the right people at the school know so that your child will be well served—while also protecting your child's privacy to the extent possible. You must balance these two competing needs.

However, you should know that school policy also dictates who at school will be notified of your child's illness—ask the school what their policy is and who will be informed as a result of it.

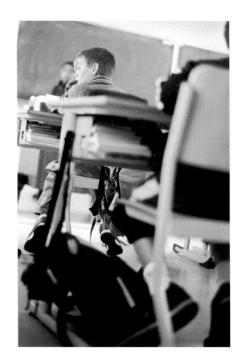

The Family Education Rights and Privacy Act of 1974 (FERPA) is a federal law that protects the privacy of school records, but under the law, faculty and staff can access the student's record if there is a legitimate academic need—so even though the privacy law exists, your child's privacy is not necessarily totally protected.

Furthermore, and understandably, under some circumstances, school personnel are **not** allowed to maintain confidentiality about your child's condition—they are required by law to report instances where they believe a child may be a danger either to himself or to others. Depending on the behavior of the child, that information may be shared within the school building, within the school district, or it may be shared with outside personnel (local law enforcement officials, the state Department of Children and Family Services or medical personnel).

What about school records? There are two types of records that the school creates for each child, both of which follow a child from school to school.

The permanent record is accessible to parents, but no one is allowed to remove information from it.

The first is called the **permanent** record. It contains report cards, attendance information, general information on school performance and a health record—height, weight and the results of screenings for vision and hearing. But it gets a bit muddy here—some schools include information about medication (particularly if the school has been asked to dispense it) or about a specific illness in the health record portion of the permanent record.

The temporary record can be accessed and parents can request that information be removed from it.

The second type of record is called a **temporary**, or sometimes **confidential**, record. This file contains IEPs and Section 504 Plans, psychological testing results, standardized test data, and all of the health information not contained in the permanent record. This information is available to parents and, unlike the permanent record, it can be excised. School policy and state (the School Records Act) and federal (FERPA) law stipulate the process.

If you wish to see your child's files and/or request that information be removed from the temporary record, ask your child's classroom teacher or advisor who you should contact. If you wish to remove information, be sure to put the request in writing. If the school refuses to remove the information, you have a right to a records hearing under both state and federal law.

Once again, though, if you are considering removing information from the temporary record, be certain to consider all sides of the issue. On the one hand, you want to protect your child's privacy. On the other hand, it's important that your child's schools have the information they need to best meet the needs of your child.

insurance

Insurance is perhaps one of the more frustrating issues for parents. It's time-consuming and often confusing.

Insurance policies differ greatly when it comes to mental health treatment—it's a good idea to have at least a basic grasp of what your insurance policy covers before you choose treatment providers for your child.

Some insurance policies do not cover mental health treatment at all. Many do, but there are often restrictions placed on the coverage. You may be limited on the number of outpatient visits you are allowed in a given time period or there may be a cap on the amount of money one person in your family can spend on mental health care. Co-payment requirements for mental disorders may be different than they are for physical illness.

Besides special restrictions on mental health coverage, you may have to deal with the usual health coverage issues. For example, if your family participates in an HMO, you will probably be restricted to a therapist approved by that particular plan in order to qualify for coverage. This, of course, may or may not be a therapist who works well with your child, or is even used to dealing with children.

Limitations on mental health coverage are common right now, but over the next year or so, you may see changes.

In October 2008, Congress passed a new law, the Mental Health Parity and Addiction Equity Act. As of January 2010, employers with 51 or more employees who provide mental health insurance to their employees must provide the same coverage for mental health treatment as they do for treatment of physical illnesses.

Between now and the time the act goes into effect, you may see revisions in your insurance coverage, so be sure to check from time to time to make sure you are taking advantage of any changes.

Testing and evaluations for your child's mental health assessment and adjustments to your child's school day may be at least partly covered by your health insurance policy.

HIPAA and privacy—Your child's privacy is protected by the Health Insurance Portability and Accountability Act of 1996 (HIPAA). HIPAA denies current and potential employers access to confidential medical records.

If you belong to a PPO, you may be able to go outside the approved list of providers to find one to your liking, but you may not get reimbursed at the same rate as if you had chosen from the approved list. Often the reimbursement rate is significantly below what you would get if you used a provider from the approved list, so it's a good idea to check with your insurance provider to see what the difference is.

Furthermore, many therapists do not participate in any insurance plans—as individual practitioners they don't have the capability to deal with the paperwork. Others limit the types of plans they will work with, generally ruling out plans that reimburse at a very low rate. This will mean that you will have the added burden of paperwork—paying the therapist yourself, submitting the claim to your health insurance provider, and following up to make sure you get reimbursed at the correct rate.

Many health insurance plans require pre-authorization for mental health claims.

Because of the confusing landscape of insurance coverage, our recommendation is that shortly after, or even before your child begins treatment, you contact your insurance company to find out coverage limits so that when you need to make treatment decisions, you know which options you will be reimbursed for and which you will not. It's not a perfect situation, but being informed about your coverage may prevent you from an unpleasant surprise down the road.

FIVE
insurance

One last thing we'd like to say about insurance. Many parents at some point during their child's treatment face having to pay out-of-pocket for treatment because their insurance coverage either doesn't cover the treatment, or their coverage has reached its limits. If this happens to you, we hope you will be able to find a way to continue your child's treatment. Talk to your

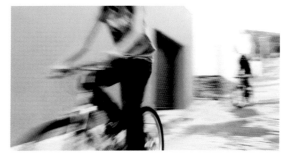

child's therapist about your financial concerns—many therapists can offer suggestions and will work with you so that your child can continue with his therapy. We believe it's important that your child get the treatment he needs—and we hope you will find a way to continue it.

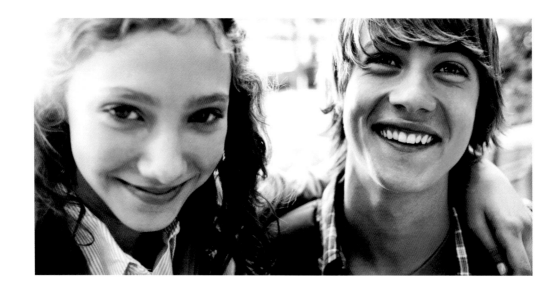

definitions and symptoms

What is depression? Depression is officially categorized as a mental disorder—that is, an illness whose symptoms are behavioral or psychological in nature as opposed to physical. Mental disorders are characterized by alterations in mood, thinking and/or behavior. Depression is an alteration of mood; thus it is classified as a mood disorder.

Note the use of the word "illness" in the definition. Mental disorders are illnesses. This has important implications—it means that we don't "cause" these disorders—and it means that treatment is often necessary for recovery, just as treatment is often necessary to recover from physical illness.

There are many different categories of mental disorders. Other than mood disorders, common mental disorders that affect children and adolescents are:
- anxiety disorders
- conduct disorder
- ADHD (attention deficit-hyperactivity disorder)
- substance-related disorders
- eating disorders
- learning disorders.

Depression in a clinical, or medical, sense has a very specific definition, at least on paper. This medical definition is designed to strike a difference between depression, the illness, and a depressed mood. Everyone feels sad sometimes—that's part of daily living— and teenagers especially feel the angst of growing up.

Major Depressive Disorder (MDD) and Major Depression (MD) are the two terms used by the medical profession for what we commonly call depression.

OFFICIAL DEFINITION OF DEPRESSION

The official definition used to diagnose depression is taken from the *DSM-IV TR* (the American Psychiatric Association's diagnostic manual). Depression, according to the manual, is the presence of at least five of the following symptoms (at least one must be either a depressed mood or loss of interest or pleasure) for at least a two-week period, and representing a change from, and impairment of, previous functioning:

- Depressed mood most of the day, nearly every day, as indicated by either subjective report (e.g., feels sad or empty) or observation made by others (e.g., appears tearful). Note: In children and adolescents, can be irritable mood.
- Markedly diminished interest or pleasure in all, or almost all, activities most of the day, nearly every day (as indicated by either subjective account or observation made by others).
- Significant weight loss when not dieting or weight gain (e.g., a change of more than 5% of body weight in a month), or decrease or increase in appetite nearly every day. Note: In children, consider failure to make expected weight gains.
- Insomnia or hypersomnia nearly every day.
- Psychomotor agitation or retardation nearly every day (observable by others, not merely subjective feelings of restlessness or being slowed down).
- Fatigue or loss of energy nearly every day.
- Feelings of worthlessness or excessive or inappropriate guilt (which may be delusional) nearly every day (not merely self-reproach or guilt about being sick).
- Diminished ability to think or concentrate, or indecisiveness, nearly every day (either by subjective account or as observed by others).
- Recurrent thoughts of death (not just fear of dying), recurrent suicidal ideation without a specific plan, or a suicide attempt or a specific plan for committing suicide.

Meeting these criteria doesn't necessarily mean a person has depression. Certain medical conditions, like thyroid disease, adrenal gland disease and diabetes, can cause many of the same symptoms. Depressive symptoms can also be a result of bereavement, alcohol abuse, street drugs or the side effects of prescription medications. All of these possibilities need to be ruled out by your child's physician or therapist before a diagnosis of depression is made.

There are varying degrees of depression: mild, moderate and severe. As you might expect, in cases of mild depression, the sufferer has sufficient symptoms for a diagnosis, but the symptoms interfere only minimally with daily life. At the opposite end of the spectrum is severe depression, in which an individual is essentially incapacitated—unable to attend school or work, even perhaps unable to get out of bed or take care of himself.

Frequent and persistent thoughts of death or suicide, or suicide attempts, are always categorized as severe depression.

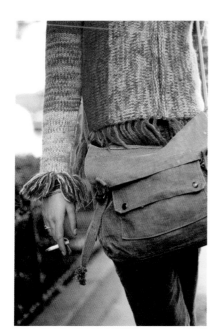

There are known risk factors for depression. These include a family history of depression or suicide, family dysfunction, prenatal damage from alcohol abuse, street drugs, medication, tobacco or other trauma, low birth weight, poverty, abuse, neglect and multiple, frequent life stressors.

However, it's important to note that these are risk factors, not definitive predictors. In other words, these conditions put a person at a higher risk for depression, but they do not cause the illness and their presence does not necessarily mean that the illness will manifest itself. In fact, researchers believe that some combination of genetic and environmental factors are responsible for triggering mental disorders like depression.

In addition to the symptoms outlined in the *DSM-IV TR*, children and adolescents who have depression frequently exhibit physical symptoms like headaches, stomach-aches and other aches and pains and they may show more socially-isolating symptoms like neglect of appearance and hygiene. Remember, though, these symptoms must be sustained over a period of weeks or months in order for there to be a diagnosis of depression.

ONE
definitions
and symptoms

The symptoms of depression vary with age. A depressed infant may show too little or too much crying, lethargy, a sad or deadpan expression, little motor activity, feeding or sleeping problems, lack of attention, lack of curiosity and a failure to grow and thrive.

Symptoms in early elementary school-aged children (ages 6 to 8) may include, in addition to the above general symptoms, poor performance in school, separation anxiety, phobias, accident-proneness and attention-seeking behavior.

It's important to note that young children are generally not able to verbalize their feelings—their depression may manifest itself with anxiety, negative behavior patterns and physical complaints.

Older elementary-schoolers and middle-schoolers (ages 9 to 12) may say they feel "stupid" or use other self-deprecating language. They may have low self-esteem and may feel unloved, and unlovable. They may be reluctant to go to school. More severe symptoms, like thoughts of suicide, sometimes appear at these ages.

Adolescents may talk about the future pessimistically. Running away, cutting or other self-injury, extreme aggressiveness, inattention to appearance, excessive risk-taking behavior and refusal to go to school are also symptoms.

Depressed children and adolescents are often irritable—and their irritability sometimes leads to aggressive behavior.

Anxiety is a frequent precursor to depression in children and adolescents. In fact, depression is frequently seen in tandem with other mental disorders. The 1999 *Mental Health: A Report of the Surgeon General* reports that two-thirds of those who suffer from

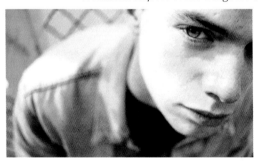

depression also suffer from another mental disorder and that, except for substance-related disorder, the depression is secondary (in other words, it arises after, and perhaps in response to, the other disorder).

The most frequent co-occurring disorders are dysthymia (defined later in this chapter), anxiety disorders, conduct disorder, substance-related disorders, ADHD (attention deficit-hyperactivity disorder) and learning disorders.

Studies tell us that in any given year, as many as 8% of our teenagers and 2.5% of our children are suffering from depression. Before age 15, depression occurs about as frequently in boys as girls; after age 15, twice as many girls suffer from it. Girls are more likely than boys to attempt suicide, but boys are more successful at completing an attempt.

Most depressive episodes last between seven and nine months. However, most people who suffer from depression will experience a relapse. Between 20% and 40% of children and adolescents will relapse within two years of a first episode, and 70% will relapse by adulthood. The relapses are usually more severe than the previous episodes.

Depression is being thought of more and more as an illness to be managed, rather than cured.

However, the news is not all bad. There is evidence to suggest that we can relieve the symptoms of depressive episodes through treatment. *A well-established base of clinical data (from real-life, as opposed to research, settings) supports the benefits of treatment, at least for short term effectiveness.*

Research on the most effective treatments for depression is ongoing. You can stay abreast of it by talking to your child's therapist and doing your own research on the Internet.

These websites have information about research currently being conducted:
- *Medlineplus.gov*
- *Healthfinder.gov*
- *Clinicaltrials.gov*
- *Nimh.nih.gov*
- *Bpkids.org*
- *Dbsalliance.org*
- *Aacap.org*
- *Narsad.org*
- *Nami.org*
- *Psychcentral.com*
- *Pdrhealth.com*

However, the scientific studies are not as definitive as the clinical evidence and so, in the end, it's difficult to draw hard, scientific conclusions about the benefits of treatment. Because of the nature of studying mental disorders like depression, especially in children and adolescents, the studies have inherent design flaws—they are generally small in sample size and of short term duration, for example. Studies of the efficacy of talk therapy are difficult because they are often conducted in research-based settings and do not translate well to real-life settings. Studies of medication are equally problematic—some of them confirm the benefits of antidepressants, for example, while others do not.

Furthermore, there are literally no studies to guide us on the efficacy or safety of long-term treatment (longer than nine months) for either talk therapy or medication, nor are there any real guides on the long-term benefits, and risks, of short-term treatments.

ONE
definitions
and symptoms

Given the confusing landscape before us, most mental health professionals today and the American Psychological Association, in its 2006 *Report of the Working Group on Psychotropic Medications for Children and Adolescents*, who reviewed all of the then-available literature, recommend a conservative approach for treating children and adolescents suffering from depression—psychotherapy first, with regular monitoring, followed by carefully controlled medication (typically one of the SSRI antidepressants) together with the psychotherapy if the psychotherapy alone is not effective. If a child is having a significant amount of trouble with daily functioning, has particularly peculiar thinking or behavior, is focused on death, has attempted suicide or is engaging in self-injurious behavior like cutting, it may be appropriate to begin with medication and psychotherapy as a combination treatment. If the situation is extremely dire—a child is an immediate threat to himself or others or if he is hearing voices or seeing things that aren't there—hospitalization may be necessary.

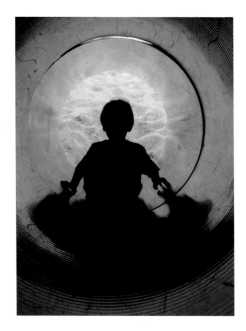

We believe that it's important for you to get help for your child if he is suffering from depression. Why? An individual with depression is at an increased risk for suicide. Ditto for substance abuse. And, as we mentioned before, 70% of children and adolescents who have a depressive episode suffer from a recurrence by adulthood. Factors that predict recurrence include the age of onset (earlier being worse), the severity and duration of the preceding episode, the number of previous episodes, the presence of other mental disorders and the presence of life stressors. Note in particular two of these factors—duration and severity; if treatment can mitigate them, then the hope is that it can reduce the occurrence and/or severity of future episodes.

For a child or adolescent suffering from depression, seven, eight or nine months is a very long time—a time when he could be getting on with the business of being a child or teenager—learning, cementing relationships and participating in the variety of activities that will help him recognize and realize his potential.

Research on the plasticity of the brain reinforces the notion that treatment is better than no treatment. The scientists who are looking at this issue hypothesize that depression somehow suppresses the brain's ability to make new brain cells—a process called neurogenesis—and that treatment corrects this, thereby promoting recovery. The brain literally rewires, and heals, itself.

OTHER MOOD DISORDERS

There are a few other mood disorders we would like to spend a little time talking about. The first is dysthymia. Dysthymia (pronounced *dis-THIGH-mee-ah*), or Dysthymic Disorder, is a mood disorder similar to mild depression, but is characterized by the fact that it lasts for at least a year, and often several years. The average duration for children and adolescents is four years. It's a tough illness—its symptoms are generally not enough to interfere significantly with a child's daily life, but they can include socially-isolating symptoms like chronic pessimism and poor social skills. And while it may not interfere with daily life, dysthymia's long duration can mean it affects normal development as much and sometimes more than depression might. Furthermore, the illness persists for so long that parents and even the child may come to believe it's just a matter of temperament—that this is the normal state of being for this child. Dysthymia puts a child at increased risk for depression; 70% eventually experience such an episode.

Bipolar disorder (sometimes referred to as manic-depressive disorder) is a complex, difficult to diagnose mood disorder. Very generally, it is characterized by cycling moods: depression followed by mania, followed by depression. The first manifestation is usually a depressive state, with the same characteristics as those of depression. The manic states are ones of persistent euphoric, expansive or irritable moods and may include inflated self-esteem, grandiosity, decreased need for sleep, talking too much or speaking too rapidly, racing or a continuous stream of thoughts, agitation, distractibility, and excessive involvement in pleasurable activities. The mania can occur just after a depressive state, months or even years afterwards, or it can occur simultaneously with the depressive state.

ONE
definitions
and symptoms

Many children and adolescents with bipolar disorder have other mental disorders as well—most commonly ADHD, conduct disorder, anxiety disorders and, particularly during adolescence, substance-related disorders.

Because the depressive states are indistinguishable from depression, and because patients in a manic state often don't recognize that they are ill or they refuse treatment, mental health professionals can have a difficult time diagnosing, much less treating, bipolar disorder. It often takes several cycles before an accurate diagnosis is made. Furthermore, bipolar disorder, because so many of its symptoms mimic ADHD (attention deficit-hyperactivity disorder), is often misdiagnosed as that, particularly in younger children (and, conversely, sometimes ADHD is misdiagnosed as bipolar disorder).

Some who suffer from bipolar disorder have a particularly intense form of the disease—rapid cycling bipolar disorder—in which sufferers can have several cycles in even one day. Children and adolescents can also suffer from mixed-state bipolar disorder, in which the depressive and manic episodes are present at the same time.

A milder form of bipolar disorder is called cyclothymia (*sigh-clo-THIGH-mee-ah*) or Cyclothymic Disorder. Cyclothymic children are kids we might call "moody" or "high-strung." They have unstable moods—cycling rapidly through periods of despair, then joy, followed by discouragement, self-confidence, and then discouragement once again, but never exhibiting the full-blown episodes of mania or depression seen in bipolar cases.

This is but a short summary of mood disorders. If your child is suffering from one of these illnesses, or any mental disorder, you may want to do more research on the Internet. Here are some websites which may be helpful:

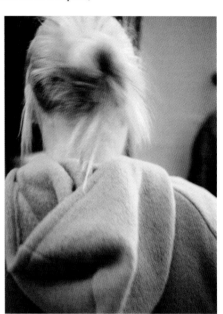

- The National Institute of Mental Health (*www.nimh.nih.gov*)
- The American Academy of Child and Adolescent Psychiatry (*www.aacap.org*)
- The American Psychological Association (*www.apa.org*)
- Mental Health America (*www.nmha.org*)
- The National Alliance on Mental Illness (*www.nami.org*)
- Mayoclinic.com
- Medlineplus.gov
- Healthfinder.gov
- Pdrhealth.com
- Psychcentral.com
- Families for Depression Awareness (*www.familyaware.org*)
- The Depression and Bipolar Support Alliance (*www.dbsalliance.org*)
- The Child and Adolescent Bipolar Foundation (*www.bpkids.org*)
- Anxiety Disorders Association of America (*www.adaa.org*)
- Obsessive-Compulsive Foundation (*www.ocfoundation.org*)
- National Eating Disorders Association (*www.nationaleatingdisorders.org*)
- Children and Adults with Attention Deficit-Hyperactivity Disorder (*www.chadd.org*).

therapists

During your child's treatment for his depression, he will work with one or more therapists—a psychiatrist, psychologist or social worker—who either practices talk therapy (psychotherapy) or prescribes medication. **Who are these people and what is their training and education?**

PSYCHIATRISTS

Psychiatrists are physicians who specialize in mental disorders. They have completed both medical school and an additional four-year residency in psychiatry. Some psychiatrists also complete a further specialty in child and adolescent psychiatry.

In addition to their formal education, most psychiatrists become certified by The American Board of Psychiatry and Neurology (*www.abpn.com*). Child and adolescent psychiatrists may be additionally certified in their specialty. Psychiatrists must be licensed by the state in which they practice.

AN IMPORTANT NOTE ABOUT HOSPITALIZATION AND THERAPISTS. Hospitals have confusing rules. Your child's therapist will not be able to see your child while he is in the hospital unless she is a staff member at the hospital or unless the attending physician at the hospital writes an order to permit it.

If your child requires hospitalization, you may want to consider taking him to the hospital where his therapist is on staff; otherwise, make sure an order is written so that she can see your child and participate in his care. Continuity of care and planning for a smooth transition home is important.

Because of their extensive training, psychiatrists have experienced an extremely broad spectrum of conditions—this can be important in the assessment and diagnosis process.

If your child needs medication for his depression, he will need to see a psychiatrist—they are the only mental health professionals who can prescribe medication. In fact, many psychiatrists do only this, and will likely be part of a team that you assemble for your child, as opposed to one therapist who will provide both the medication and talk therapy parts of the treatment.

Psychiatrists generally work in private practice, university-affiliated clinics and at hospitals.

PSYCHOLOGISTS AND SOCIAL WORKERS

Psychologists. There are different kinds of psychologists—those who practice therapy are called clinical psychologists. (Experimental, cognitive and social psychologists focus on research, developmental psychologists work with very young children who are not developing normally and school psychologists focus on testing and evaluation for learning disorders.)

Clinical psychologists hold a degree in psychology—at least a master's degree and usually a Ph.D. (doctor of philosophy) or a Psy.D. (doctor of psychology). In addition, clinical psychologists must have completed some period of time, usually two years, of supervised clinical practice and must be licensed by the state in which they practice. Clinical psychologists can become certified by the American Board of Professional Psychology (*www.abpp.org*) and some obtain additional certification in specialties such as clinical psychology, child and adolescent psychology, neuropsychology and cognitive and behavioral psychology.

It's important once again to note that there is a difference between clinical psychologists, who practice individual therapy, and school psychologists, whose expertise is in school testing and evaluations. We emphasize this distinction because people sometimes confuse the two. If your child is seeing the psychologist at his school, those sessions are specifically aimed at issues related to learning and the school environment. The services offered by therapists outside of the school are very different—they offer the therapy needed to treat your child for his illness.

Social workers. Like clinical psychologists, clinical social workers (sometimes called psychiatric social workers) practice talk therapy—but their university degree is in social work. Most clinical social workers have at least a master's degree (M.S.W.) and sometimes they have a doctorate (D.S.W. or Ph.D.). Both of these degrees require supervised clinical work. Social workers can become certified by the National Association of Social Workers (*www.socialworkers.org*). The most common certification is the A.C.S.W., which is the general certification, but there are many specialty certifications, including ones for working with children and adolescents. In addition, social workers must be licensed by the state in which they work. The commonly seen letters L.C.S.W. signify that a social worker has been licensed by the state.

As we said before, the role of the psychologist or social worker is talk therapy. What's the difference between these two professionals? Mostly their education. A psychologist's education is in the broad field of psychology—the study of human behavior. A social work degree focuses more on the interactions of individuals and groups. Having said that, the distinction may not be particularly useful in choosing one over the other when you are selecting your child's therapist—both are required to spend time in supervised clinical settings in order to be certified and licensed to practice therapy. In the end, it's really most important to choose someone who:

Although they cannot prescribe and monitor medication, many psychologists and social workers work with clients who take medication for their depression. Your child's psychologist or social worker may be a good sounding board for you to determine whether or not his medication is working well, and whether there are other alternatives.

- has a formal education and the proper training to be a qualified therapist
- has a broad range of experience
- works well with your child.

In addition, because different therapists practice different types of therapies (which are discussed in the next chapter), it's important that you know which type of therapy your child's therapist practices—and that this type of therapy meets the needs of your child.

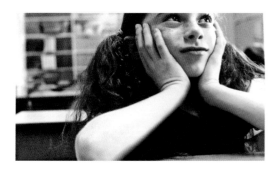

One important note of difference between a clinical psychologist and social worker is that clinical psychologists, like psychiatrists, generally have more expertise in assessment than do social workers. You may want to consider this difference when choosing someone to do your child's initial mental health assessment.

Psychologists and social workers generally work as solo practitioners in private practice, or with other therapists in a group practice. They can also be found at local social service agencies. Very often these agencies are a gateway for people who need help. Hospitals also often have psychologists and social workers as part of their mental health staff, especially in their clinics. Police departments and schools also often employ social workers and psychologists (remember, however, that they may not be trained for clinical practice) and these people are often the first people who see children and adolescents who are in crisis—they often have a wealth of information about local services.

TWO
therapists

OTHER KINDS OF THERAPISTS OR COUNSELORS

There are other kinds of therapists or counselors you may be referred to during the course of your child's treatment: art therapists, marriage and family therapists and various types of counselors are among the list.

Art therapists, as the name implies, use art as an expression of emotion and may be particularly useful for younger children or those who have a difficult time verbalizing their thoughts and feelings.

A marriage and family therapist (M.F.T. or L.M.F.T.) may also be appropriate for your child or family. Marriage and family therapists specialize in family dynamics. They treat both individuals and families by focusing on family relationships and the issues that are causing discord in the family.

Counselors are people who offer advice or guidance (as opposed to psychotherapy, which by definition is a therapy to treat a disorder). Churches, for example, often have pastoral counselors, and schools often employ school counselors. Addiction counselors help people with their addiction.

Many of these therapists and counselors have attended an accredited program to train them in their practice and many are licensed by the state. However, some are not. Hopefully, the person who referred you to a particular therapist or counselor knows the background and credentials of the person she referred you to, but you should also check credentials and references.

In Illinois, you can check to see whether your child's therapist or counselor is licensed by going to the Illinois Department of Financial and Professional Regulation's website at *www.idfpr.com*. Click on "License Look-up Information."

talk therapy

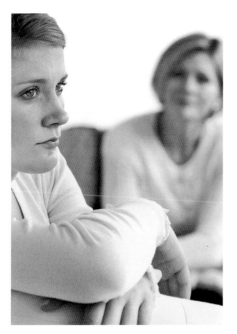

Has anyone on the planet not heard of Freud and his impact on how we see ourselves and others? It's really quite profound, and we have much to thank Freud for. However, psychotherapy has changed a lot in the past few decades—it is no longer the familiar "Freudian" psychoanalysis that has Woody Allen lying on the couch in the therapist's office talking about his mother.

The advent of psychotropic drugs in the 1970s was a watershed event. These drugs changed the way we looked at mental disorders—the very fact that they worked forced us to consider that mental disorders are at least partly biologically based and not solely a result of past experiences. Because of this, therapists began to explore new kinds of talk therapies—therapies aimed more at helping patients change their behaviors than analyzing past experiences and memories. Their focus was less on the "why," but rather on helping patients in a very practical way to change their belief systems and behaviors; they are more rooted in the present than the past.

Many therapies today blend the two viewpoints, borrowing some techniques from the newer "behavior modification" trends and some from the more traditional "analysis" therapies. Therapy for children and adolescents in particular tends to be focused on the "behavior modification" end of the spectrum—children have less of a past to analyze.

We can summarize (and it is a summary indeed) the kinds of therapy that are most commonly practiced today into three basic types: psychodynamic psychotherapy, cognitive behavioral therapy and interpersonal therapy.

COMMON KINDS OF THERAPY

Psychodynamic psychotherapy. Psychodynamic psychotherapy (also called dynamic psychotherapy, psychoanalytic psychotherapy, insight-oriented psychotherapy or exploratory psychotherapy) is perhaps closest to what we think of as traditional Freudian therapy. Psychodynamic psychotherapy aims at helping patients discover the unconscious source of their mental disorder. It often focuses on childhood experiences and repressed memories— discovering the root of the problem allows the patient to "let go" of his negative feelings and behaviors. Psychodynamic psychotherapy is not the mainstay therapy today, but some therapists use it occasionally during therapy sessions when they see the need for deeper analysis of motives and behaviors.

Cognitive behavioral therapy. Cognitive behavioral therapy (CBT) is on the other end of the continuum from psychodynamic psychotherapy. It is a time-limited, practical, problem-focused approach in which the patient literally works to retrain his thinking. It is aimed at helping the patient understand that his distorted beliefs about himself and the world lead to negative feelings and then to counterproductive behaviors, which cycle back to reinforce his distorted belief system. If he can break one link in the chain, the cycle is broken, the distorted beliefs are corrected and the symptoms are reduced in a process called "cognitive restructuring." CBT, or some derivative of it, is probably the most commonly practiced form of psychotherapy today.

Interpersonal therapy. Interpersonal therapy (IPT) focuses on improving the patient's interactions with others. Like CBT, there is less focus on the "why" of behaviors or on the past; rather the focus is on the now and on practical strategies for helping the patient problem-solve and improve his relationships, and thereby feel better about himself. Because of its emphasis on relationships, IPT (in a form specifically designed for adolescents called IPT-A, or Interpersonal Therapy for Adolescents) is sometimes used for adolescents, when peer and parent relationships are so very important.

CBT and IPT-A are the only two forms of talk therapy that have been systematically studied in adolescents. These studies generally (though not always) confirm the benefits of both treatments for the short term. However, it is worthwhile to note that a particular drawback of most studies is that they are conducted at university clinics, where the therapists are highly trained in the therapy being tested. Generally, once therapies are used in real-life settings, effectiveness decreases, arguing for making sure your child's therapist is well-trained. The data on the long-term efficacy of either of these therapies are not sufficient to draw any conclusions from.

Even though talk therapies like CBT and IPT are time-limited, repeated courses may be needed to address relapses of your child's illness.

Having said that, however, we are reminded that clinical evidence and a consensus in the mental health community support the use of both CBT and IPT/IPT-A for treating depression in adolescents.

Neither CBT or IPT/IPT-A have been well studied in children. In fact, some therapists believe that cognitive approaches are more difficult for this age group because children are not ready for these higher-level thinking activities.

OTHER KINDS OF THERAPY

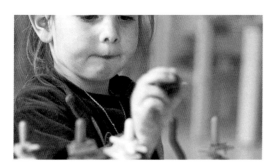

There are other kinds of therapies—non-directive supportive therapy, dialectical behavior therapy, narrative therapy, animal therapy, eye movement desensensitization and reprocessing (EMDR), etc.—that you may run across, but none have been well studied. Many websites explain these newer therapies—at the end of this handbook we have a list of websites that may be able to help you understand any therapies your child's therapist recommends.

There are also therapeutic techniques that your child's therapist may use from time to time, or even most of the time, during therapy sessions—play, movement and art therapy are three of them. These techniques can help your child's therapist understand your child's emotional state in non-verbal ways—which may be particularly appropriate for younger children or children and adolescents who have a difficult time verbalizing their thoughts and feelings.

THREE
talk therapy

Psychoeducation is a word you might hear about, too. It is being used more and more as an adjunct to any treatment of depression. Psychoeducation is simply educating the patient and his family about depression. From a common sense standpoint, psychoeducation seems like a good idea. The more we can learn about an illness, the more we can understand and relate to the family member who is suffering—and that can only be a good thing. It should be a normal part of all therapy.

Group and Family Therapies. In addition to the individual therapies above, group therapy is a common form of therapy practiced today, particularly when a patient's issues are part of the dynamics of the family or a peer group. There are two basic types of group therapy—family therapy and peer-to-peer group therapy.

If your child is in individual therapy, you, other family members and/or your child may be asked to attend family therapy sessions. The goal of family therapy (sometimes practiced in specific forms knows as systemic family therapy or multi-systemic family therapy) is to change the dynamics in a family—sometimes family dynamics can contribute to one member's depression and sometimes one member's depression can set in motion a family dynamic that impacts everyone in a negative way.

While it is often recommended, there is not sufficient research to draw any conclusions about the efficacy of family therapy for children or adolescents with depression. However, we would make the point that common sense argues that one family member's mood and behavior affects everyone in the family, and, at the very least, if everyone has an opportunity in a safe setting to express their emotions and gain some understanding about one another's feelings, that is a good thing. Also, having the entire family in therapy may help the child who is suffering from depression—if everyone is going to therapy, he may not feel so alone, so different.

Peer-to-peer group therapy is most often used in hospital settings or day programs where patients work together to solve common problems. It's a meeting-type format in which the therapist acts as a facilitator. It's usually used to address one particular issue, for example substance abuse, or to help children build and practice social skills. It's thought that these types of issues are more effectively addressed with one's peers than individually with one's therapist, though, again, there is not sufficient research to know whether it is an effective tool for either children or adolescents.

medications

The decision to use medication to treat your child's or adolescent's depression is a difficult one. The research is confusing and inconclusive. The very subject matter is difficult to study—subjective symptoms like mood, thoughts and behavior don't easily lend themselves to objective measure. In addition, there are ethical issues when it comes to studying any illness in children and adolescents.

Because of these kinds of inherent problems, we don't have the kind of information about whether and how to treat mental disorders in children and adolescents with medication that we would like to have; the studies we have are few in number, small in size and limited in scope.

One concern is that the studies only assess short term efficacy—they tell us nothing about either long term efficacy or safety. Another problem is that, although there are many medications to treat depression on the market, only one such medication, fluoxetine (brand name Prozac), has been approved by the FDA for use in children and adolescents, and most of the studies we have for children and adolescents focus solely on that medication. Other medications, which are often used "off label" to treat children and adolescents, have much less research behind them to support their use. And studies on the use of medication in younger children are virtually non-existent.

Physicians prescribe a medication "off label" to a patient when they believe the medication will help alleviate symptoms, even though the medication hasn't been approved by the FDA for that particular illness or it hasn't been approved for use in the patient's age group. Ironically, "off label" prescribing occurs frequently for children and adolescents (for all medication, not just psychotropic medication) because of the ethical concerns about conducting studies on these age groups.

All of this leaves physicians and parents with not much information (other than informed experience in the case of physicians) to help them make a decision about whether to treat a child's depression with medication and which medication to use. However, despite the lack of solid scientific evidence supporting the use of medication, many mental health professionals and parents advocate for its use.

In addition to clinical evidence that medication works, they point to one important statistic—overall suicide rates for children and adolescents have decreased since the advent of antidepressants, at a time when rates of depression have not decreased commensurately, suggesting, but not proving, a cause-and-effect relationship between the two.

CONSIDERING MEDICATION

Given all this, how do we, as parents, consider the options when thinking about giving our children medication to treat their depression? In the end, it's a good question, with a not very good answer. It boils down to trusting your child's psychiatrist, being as informed as you can, rigorously monitoring your child (both the taking of the medication and its effects and side effects) and keeping a bit of an open mind about both trying, adjusting or discontinuing the use of medication if benefits are not seen, or if the side effects are significant.

BLACK BOX WARNING ON ANTIDEPRESSANTS.
One much-discussed side effect of antidepressant use is suicidal ideation (thinking about suicide). In 2004, the FDA issued a "black box warning" that the use of antidepressants in children, adolescents and young adults could lead to increased thoughts of suicide. It should be noted that while an increase in suicidal ideation did occur in the studies cited in the warning, in fact, no actual suicides occurred.

The warning reinforces the need for careful monitoring of antidepressant medication. If your child is prescribed an antidepressant, make sure that you and his psychiatrist are watching closely for signs of suicidal thinking or attempts.

We have said it before, and we will say it again. Most mental health professionals and The American Psychological Association, in its 2006 *Report of the Working Group on Psychotropic Medications for Children and Adolescents*, recommend a conservative approach when treating children and adolescents for depression—psychotherapy first, with regular monitoring, followed by carefully controlled medication (typically one of the SSRI antidepressants) together with the psychotherapy if the psychotherapy alone is not effective. If, however, your child is having significant difficulty with daily functioning, has particularly peculiar thinking, is focused on death, has attempted suicide or is engaging in other self-injurious behavior such as cutting, it may be best to begin with medication and psychotherapy as a combination treatment. If the situation is extremely dire—if your child is an immediate threat to himself or others or if he is hearing voices or seeing things that aren't there—you may need to consider hospitalization.

So, with this very complicated picture before us, we turn to the medication itself and some things you should know if you make the decision to begin medication.

First and foremost, you should know that medication doesn't cure a mental disorder—it alleviates the symptoms, hopefully helping your child to function, participate in talk therapy, connect with other people, and ultimately recover from his episode.

Secondly, illnesses like depression and bipolar disorder are complicated and our bodies are equally complicated. What works for one person doesn't work for another—it's the rule rather than the exception that a lot of tweaking of psychotropic medication, both the type of medication and the dose, is required to find the one that works, in the dose that works. In addition, several medications may be needed to fully address your child's illness, or an additional medication may be needed to address the negative side effects of the first medication.

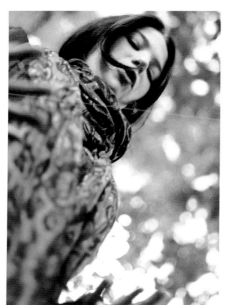

Finally, children, adolescents and adults all metabolize medication differently. Younger people generally absorb medications into the blood stream more rapidly than older people do—this can cause higher peaking and more immediate side effects in children and adolescents than in adults. And younger people eliminate medications differently than adults do. A child's liver is proportionately larger than an adult's, so it eliminates medications more rapidly. Furthermore, many of these medications are absorbed into fat tissue before being released into the blood stream for use, which, especially for adolescent girls, can vary significantly over very short periods of time.

All of this means that the prescribing psychiatrist must consider a wide variety of factors when she chooses which medication and which dose best suits your child—and it means that there may be continuous need for adjustments before she finds the right medication and the right dose for your child. The general rule of thumb is to begin with the lowest dose possible, and then increase in small doses thereafter until the medication becomes effective.

FOUR
medications

SIDE EFFECTS

The problem of side effects can be an issue for your child. Many of the most common side effects occur shortly after beginning the medication and disappear within a few weeks. But some side effects are long term—often they can be managed by adjusting dosages or medications, but not always. The issue of side effects is further complicated by the age of your child—younger children may not be able to articulate what they are feeling.

Some initial side effects, particularly suicidal ideation, can be dangerous. For that reason, it's important that your child see his psychiatrist frequently at the beginning of the process and whenever

Many psychotropic medications can be toxic and it's not always easy to tell what dose will be toxic for one person versus another. Some people inherently metabolize medications more slowly than others. In addition, several medications are sometimes required and the medications can interact with one another.

We will say it again—your child's psychiatrist should monitor any psychotropic medication your child is taking.

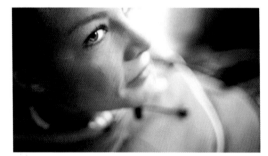

doses are adjusted or new medications are tried. The FDA recommends that your child see his psychiatrist for regular monitoring once a week during the first month of treatment and every two weeks during the second month. Regular monitoring, at least monthly, after that should occur.

The problem of long term side effects is a real issue. We don't know much about whether there are serious long-term side effects from even short-term use of psychotropic medication taken by children and adolescents. More research in this area is sorely needed.

Most psychotropic medications, antidepressant medications in particular, take time to work—up to four to six weeks—and even then relief from symptoms may be gradual. Furthermore, psychotropic medications tend to lose their effectiveness over time, so you may find that after a period of months, the medication that worked for your child no longer does and you have to go back to the drawing board. It can be frustrating for you and your child, but know that it is a normal part of using these medications.

In addition, psychotropic medications can have a significant impact on other medications, even over-the-counter medications, being taken. Careful monitoring and complete disclosure to all of your child's physicians of medications (including over-the-counter medications, vitamins, herbal remedies and recreational drugs/alcohol) is a must. Most psychotropic medications should not be taken with alcohol or other recreational drugs; this issue should be thoroughly discussed with your child and his psychiatrist, especially if your child has a history of alcohol or drug use.

Children should not be responsible for taking psychotropic medication and all children and adolescents should be monitored when they take psychotropic medication.

Taking medication for mental disorders can be a pretty hard thing for your child. When he first begins a medication, the side effects can be annoying—nausea, diarrhea, dry mouth, sleep disturbances, weight gain, the list can be extensive—and taking medication for a mental disorder can make one feel ashamed. It's important to establish an open attitude with your child about taking his medication and remind him that many of these annoying symptoms will subside in a few weeks. It may be helpful to compare taking psychotropic medication to taking medication for other kinds of medical problems, like an antibiotic for an ear infection, for example. You can tell your child that it's supposed to help him feel better (though it might take some time before it takes effect), and he deserves to do just that—feel better.

It's also pretty common for children and adolescents (and adults) to forget to take their medication, or to decide that they don't need it any more. This is particularly true once the medication begins to be effective. But withdrawal from these medications can be very difficult, and even dangerous, so it's important that your child know how important it is to continue to take his medication on a daily basis, at the same time of day, and to continue his medication, even if he thinks he doesn't really need it. The medication journal can be helpful here—check it from time to time.

Withdrawal from psychotropic medication can be severe. You or your child should not make the unilateral decision to stop his medication. When it's time for your child to stop taking his medication, it is very important that your child taper down from using medication gradually, and under the supervision of his psychiatrist.

You can also check to make sure whether your child is taking his medication by keeping track of how many pills are in the bottle—if there are too many pills in it, then your child is not taking his medication. We should mention that it is not unheard of for children and adolescents to flush their medication down the toilet or otherwise dispose of it, or even sell or give it to others, so be careful about using the bottle check as your only evidence that your child is taking his medication. It's really best to have your child take his medication in your presence.

FOUR
medications

All of this at a time when your child is suffering is a lot to deal with. There are no easy answers when contemplating the use of medication to treat your child's depression. The best we can do is to recommend a long discussion with everyone involved to decide what's best—as we said before, there are times when the benefits of taking medication outweigh all of the potential risks and side effects and there are times when it's better to proceed with talk therapy and hold off on the medication.

PSYCHOTROPIC MEDICATIONS

There are four classes of psychotropic medications used to treat mood disorders:
- antidepressants
- mood stabilizers
- antipsychotics
- antianxiety medications.

In general, antidepressants are by far the most used psychotropic medications and are used for the most common mood disorder—depression. Mood stabilizers are used for the treatment of bipolar disorder and sometimes as a secondary medication for depression. Antipsychotic medications are sometimes used to treat bipolar disorder or as short-term fast-acting medications for very severe episodes of depression. Antianxiety medications are used, as the name suggests, for the treatment of anxiety disorders—panic disorders, phobias, obsessive compulsive disorder (OCD), etc.—which often accompany depression.

Finally, though this is not a treatise on ADHD (attention deficit-hyperactivity disorder), we should mention the ADHD medications—particularly stimulants (Ritalin, Adderall, Concerta, etc.). Much is written, and debated, about the use of these medications. This handbook is not intended to address the complicated issue of ADHD, but we do recognize that many children with ADHD frequently also have other mental disorders, including depression. Given the complicated landscape of medications for both illnesses, we can only advise you to make certain that any prescribing physician is aware of which medications your child is taking, and that she is qualified to understand the implications of simultaneously medicating your child for both disorders.

With this backdrop of information in mind, we will now discuss each of the classes of medications in more detail.

ANTIDEPRESSANTS

Researchers speculate that depression is in some way linked to substances in the body called neurotransmitters. There are over two hundred different neurotransmitters in the body—the ones you are probably familiar with are dopamine, norepinephrine and serotonin.

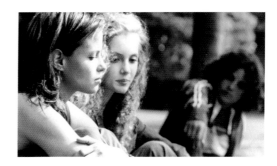

Neurotransmitters reside in neurons, the cells that constitute the nervous system—their job is to help transmit information from one neuron to another so that the body can act and react.

The most well known antidepressants are called re-uptake inhibitors. This class of drugs literally stops, or "inhibits," the absorption, or "re-uptake," of neurotransmitters from the synapse, or end, of a neuron, where they are active, back into the interior of the neuron, where they become inactive. Thus, re-uptake inhibitors have the effect of increasing the level of neurotransmitters that are active in the body. Some re-uptake inhibitors target one neurotransmitter, most commonly serotonin; others target more than one. Researchers believe that depression is the result of a complex interplay between many different neurotransmitters.

A REMINDER: It's important that if your child is taking medication for his depression that he continue with his talk therapy. The two treatments complement one another. It's also important that the psychiatrist who prescribes the medication and the talk therapist communicate frequently so that appropriate adjustments can be made to your child's treatment plan. It is often up to the parent to make sure this happens—busy therapists often overlook this critical step in the process.

Re-uptake inhibitors have been around since the 1960s. The first class of re-uptake inhibitors to be developed works on the neurotransmitters norepinephrine and, to a lesser extent, serotonin. These re-uptake inhibitors are called tricyclic antidepressants, TCAs (because of the three rings in their chemical structure).

Tricyclics are not used much anymore because there are newer classes of re-uptake inhibitors with less severe side effects—overdoses of tricyclics can be very dangerous. However, they are still used occasionally, sometimes to treat ADHD, tic disorders, obsessive-compulsive disorder and bed-wetting in children and adolescents. In general, studies have shown that tricyclics are not effective for treating depression in children and adolescents.

FOUR
medications

The newer, and most widely prescribed, classes of antidepressants are known by their acronyms—SSRIs, SNRIs, NRIs, NASSAs, etc. The most well known, and most used, are the SSRIs—selective serotonin re-uptake inhibitors. As you may guess, SSRIs work to increase active levels of serotonin. The other acronyms vary by the specific neurotransmitter(s) that they target, but are usually referred to as second or third generation (or atypical) antidepressants to relieve the acronym confusion.

There are many of these medications on the market today and if your child needs medication to help him with his depression, he will probably begin with this class of antidepressants. They include:

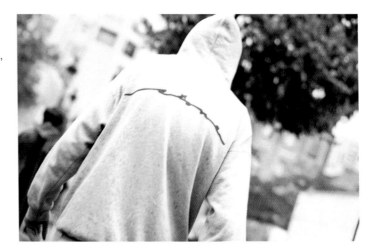

- fluoxetine (Prozac)
- sertraline (Zoloft)
- escitalopram (Lexapro)
- citalopram (Celexa)
- fluvoxamine (Luvox)
- bupropion (Wellbutrin)
- duloxetine (Cymbalta)
- mirtazapine (Remeron)
- venlafaxine (Effexor)
- paroxetine (Paxil, Pexeva).

Fluoxetine (Prozac) is the only antidepressant medication approved by the FDA to treat depression in children and adolescents aged 8 and older.

Like most medications, antidepressants have side effects. Some are present during the first few weeks of taking the medication and then subside, and some are more persistent. The list is long and can include headache, nausea, gastrointestinal problems, diarrhea, constipation, vomiting, nervousness, agitation, skin rash, sleep problems, drowsiness, change in appetite, dizziness, irritability, blunting of emotions, weight gain, a feeling of being "wired" or over-stimulated and decreased sexual libido.

Some side effects can be controlled through adjustment of the dosage, but some cannot. On occasion, antidepressants, as with other psychotropic medications, can have the reverse effect—they exacerbate the depression that they are intended to alleviate. There are also reports that antidepressants may suppress growth, though this has not been confirmed.

Side effects vary significantly by individual and the only way to know which side effects your child may experience is informed trial and error, based on your child's psychiatrist's experience in general and with patients similar to your child.

Antidepressants require regular monitoring for side effects. Side effects and medical risks often increase when antidepressants are combined with other medications—in particular, negative interactions can occur when taking antidepressants with some antihistamines, antibiotics, blood pressure medications, stimulants, pain medications, sedatives and mood stabilizers.

Withdrawal from antidepressants can be difficult, including increased risk for manic episodes. Discontinuing their use requires tapering down the doses over a period of time and must be monitored by your child's psychiatrist.

Finally, we are again reminded that it's important to get a proper diagnosis when contemplating the use of an antidepressant for your child. Using antidepressants for people with bipolar disorder may provoke a manic episode or cause a spike in mood, leading to a bigger, potentially more dangerous drop afterward. It's very important to have an accurate diagnosis of your child's illness and to be careful to note any unusual behaviors while taking antidepressants.

Another class of antidepressants works differently than those listed above. These antidepressants are called monoamine oxidase inhibitors (MAOIs). These medications also increase the level of neurotransmitters in the body, but in a different way—they inactivate an enzyme in the body that is responsible for metabolizing them. MAOIs have significant obstacles to use—many common foods interact dangerously with them— and so they are generally only used as a last line of defense for treating depression. MAOIs are not approved for use in children or adolescents.

MOOD STABILIZERS

Mood stabilizers, also called antimanic medications, are medications that even out, or stabilize, one's mood. They are used, often in conjunction with one another, to treat bipolar disorder and are sometimes used together with antidepressants to treat depression.

One of the most commonly used mood stabilizers is lithium. It has been used for fifty years to treat bipolar disorder and a significant body of knowledge has grown up around it to help guide its administration and monitoring. Lithium is approved by the FDA for treating bipolar disorder in children aged 12 and older.

Research on the best treatment protocol for bipolar disorder is ongoing. In March 2005, the *Journal of the American Academy of Child and Adolescent Psychiatry* published treatment guidelines for children and adolescents with bipolar disorder. These guidelines are available at the Academy's website at *www.aacap.org*.

Lithium is extremely dose-sensitive, so it must be carefully administered and regularly monitored. It can adversely affect the thyroid and kidneys.

Lithium has a fairly wide range of side effects, particularly when first taking it, including restlessness, mental slowing, drowsiness, weakness, fatigue, nausea, diarrhea, gastrointestinal problems, hair loss or thinning, weight gain, tremors, acne flare-ups, hypothyroidism, dry mouth, excessive thirst, water retention and increased urination (including bed-wetting in children). Many of these side effects can be managed by adjusting the dosage. Longer term side effects can include weakened bones, weight gain, hypothyroidism and kidney damage. In addition, birth defects are associated with the use of lithium if used during pregnancy and caution should be taken when using lithium during breast-feeding.

Be sure to ask your child's psychiatrist about the symptoms that signal toxic levels of lithium. The list is fairly long—you should be aware of them and call your child's psychiatrist immediately if any should develop.

Because of the way lithium works in the body, sodium levels are important—both significant increases and decreases can be dangerous. If your child is taking lithium, he should be careful not to increase or reduce his sodium intake excessively—even drinking too much or too little water, sweating, vomiting or diarrhea, the use of diuretics, or crash dieting can be dangerous. Also, you should be careful about the regular use of some anti-inflammatory agents (such as ibuprofen) and excessive intake of caffeine when taking lithium.

The other mood stabilizers that are used to treat bipolar disorder are the group of medications known as anticonvulsants. Because of the dose-sensitivity of lithium, and because lithium does not work for everyone, this class of medications, originally designed to prevent seizures, is being used more and more as an alternative to lithium.

The anticonvulsant valproate, divalproex or valproic acid (Depacon, Depakote, Depakene and Stavzor) is the most commonly used anticonvulsant medication to treat bipolar disorder—used probably as much as lithium, especially to treat rapid-cycling bipolar disorder.

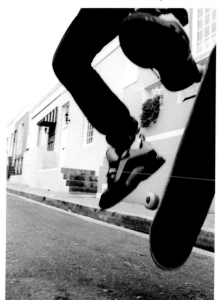

As with other psychotropic medications, valproate has a long list of potential side effects. Initial side effects can include gastrointestinal upset, headache, dizziness, double vision, anxiety, confusion and sleepiness. More long-lasting side effects are increased appetite, weight gain, tremors and hair loss. In addition, there is a chance of birth defects associated with the use of valproate during pregnancy and caution should be taken when using it during breast-feeding. Valproate can also cause cessation of menstruation, excess facial and body hair and ovarian cysts in teenage girls and women.

The dosage of this medication varies greatly from person to person depending on metabolism rates—regular monitoring is required to check for liver and pancreatic toxicity. Talk to your child's psychiatrist about the symptoms that signal toxicity.

Valproate has not been approved by the FDA for use in children or adolescents for bipolar disorder, though it has been approved to treat bipolar disorder in adults.

There are other anticonvulsants used to treat bipolar disorder, though they are used less frequently than lithium and valproate. These include carbamazepine (Tegretol), lamotrigine (Lamictal), gabapentin (Neurontin), oxcarbazepine (Trileptal), topiramate (Topamax), and tiagabine (Gabitril). As with other psychotropic medication, the side effects of these medications can be significant. None have been approved for treating bipolar disorder in children and adolescents. As with valproate, regular monitoring should be done to check for toxicity.

FOUR
medications

ANTIPSYCHOTICS

If your child is having a particularly severe episode of depression, has delusions or hallucinations, or is in need of hospitalization, you may find yourself being asked to consider an antipsychotic medication. Because antipsychotic drugs act rapidly to relieve symptoms, they are used to bridge the gap between the onset of taking an antidepressant and when it begins to take effect.

Antipsychotics are also used as a stand-alone medication to treat bipolar disorder in children and adolescents if other medications have failed to be effective and are also sometimes used early on to level out a manic episode until a mood stabilizer takes effect.

Like re-uptake inhibitors, antipsychotic drugs have gone through a generation since their discovery in the 1950s. The class of antipsychotic drugs used today is called "atypical antipsychotics." Included in this class of medications are risperidone (Risperdal), olanzapine (Zyprexa), quetiapine (Seroquel), aripiprazole (Abilify), ziprasidone (Geodon), and clozapine (Clozaril). These medications have not been approved by the FDA for children younger than 18.

If your child is asked to take an antipsychotic medication, it's a good idea to do some research on the specific type of medication he is being asked to take. The side effects, especially the long-term ones, of these medications can be serious, and include increased risk of diabetes and cardiovascular disease (both of which should be monitored for regularly). Your child's psychiatrist and research on the Internet can give you specific information about the risks and benefits of these medications. We have a listing of several on-line resources at the end of this chapter.

ANTIANXIETY MEDICATIONS

If your child suffers from an anxiety disorder, he may be asked to take an antianxiety medication. While antidepressants can be effective to treat anxiety disorders and are often used to do so, antianxiety medications are specifically designed to treat anxiety, and they relieve symptoms quickly.

Antianxiety medications include the benzodiazepines such as clonazepam (Klonopin), alprazolam (Xanax), diazepam (Valium), lorezapam (Ativan) and triazolam (Halcion). Their side effects include sleepiness, loss of coordination, fatigue and mental slowing. For some people, these medications can have the opposite effect—they can increase anxiety rather than relieve it.

These drugs can be habit-forming—abuse of them can easily occur and sudden withdrawal can be dangerous. Because of this, they are most often used on a temporary or an as-needed basis. These medications have not been approved for use in children younger than 18 years old.

The other drug used to treat anxiety and sometimes as a secondary medication for depression is buspirone (BuSpar). It is not a fast-acting medication, cannot be taken on an as-needed basis as can the benzodiazepines listed above, and is not generally as effective as the benzodiazepines—but it does not have the same risk of addiction or dependence. Side effects include dizziness, drowsiness, nausea, headache and nervousness. BuSpar has not been approved for use in children and adolescents under the age of 18.

MORE INFORMATION ON MEDICATION

This section on medication has been only a starter for you. There is much more information you will want to ask your child's psychiatrist about—she should be able to answer many, if not all, of your questions.

In addition, there is a plethora of information on the Internet—of course the usual precautions should be taken when relying on information you get from the Internet, but here are some websites you may want to refer to:

Information about psychotropic medications changes relatively frequently. It's a good idea to check with your child's psychiatrist from time to time to see whether there is any new information that would suggest discontinuance of your child's medication or whether there is any reason to believe that a different medication might be more effective for your child. You may also want to ask to see the research or to read about it online.

- The Food and Drug Administration (*www.fda.gov*)
- The National Institute of Mental Health (*www.nimh.nih.gov*)
- The American Academy of Child and Adolescent Psychiatry (*www.aacap.org*)
- Medlineplus.gov
- Pdrhealth.com
- Mayoclinic.com
- Psychcentral.com
- Drugs.com.

FOUR
medications

other treatments

Like any other difficult, chronic illness, when it comes to mental disorders like depression, there is a plethora of alternative treatments available, almost jumping out at you, to consider. Some of them are silly, and some are commonsensical. Some will seem too good to be true—and probably are. This chapter is written to give you a general, very general, sense of some of the alternatives being discussed today.

We will begin with the commonsensical—treatments that are just good for you anyway and that your child can put into practice right away.

There is good evidence to support regular, vigorous exercise to alleviate the symptoms of depression, especially mild depression. Researchers believe that exercise works on the brain much in the same way as antidepressants do—it promotes the growth, or neurogenesis, of new brain cells.

The April 2008 issue of the *Harvard Health Letter* states that "some research has shown that a fairly strenuous exercise program results in a 50% decrease in depressive symptoms … Physical activity may affect the brain directly by boosting neurogenesis: brain cells grow a bit and make more connections where it counts."

And, we all know that a healthy diet has all kinds of benefits, and it may help with depression. Encourage your child to eat a good diet, rich in fruits, vegetables, legumes, whole grains and low-fat proteins and limit sugar, simple carbohydrates (white bread, pasta, white rice), and, of course, avoid alcohol, tobacco and street drugs.

Also, an established routine, with regular bedtime and sufficient sleep is critical. Sleep researchers who look at the brain images of sleep-deprived individuals see similarities between this group of people and those who are suffering from depression. Adolescents need at least nine hours of sleep a night, and many of them are getting far less than that.

The bottom line is: encourage your child to do these things—they may help him feel better. But, remember, even though it goes without saying that these things are wise for anyone to practice, they can be just more things undone and more to feel guilty about when one

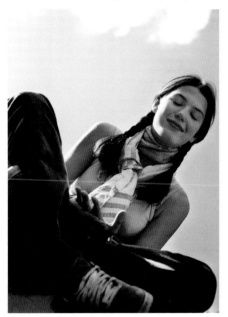

is depressed, so don't be alarmed if your child doesn't want to or can't participate in these healthy activities. Be patient—it may be that your child needs to get into treatment for a while and get a little better before he has the energy and interest to add these things to his daily routine.

There is some evidence that omega-3 fatty acids (found in fish oil) may help with milder forms of depression. As this book goes to press, there is an ongoing clinical trial on the effect of omega-3 fatty acids to treat depression in adolescents. There is also some suggestion that B vitamins are helpful—there is a study being conducted now on the impact of Vitamin B-9, folic acid.

There is evidence to suggest that meditation, breathing exercises and yoga may help relieve the symptoms of depression. Some research has shown that meditation literally changes the brain— people who meditate show physical increases in the size of and activity in the part of the cortex associated with emotions.

Many people experiment with treatments such as acupuncture, massage, relaxation techniques and full-spectrum light therapy. In fact, some of these treatments are recommended by therapists as adjunct treatments to medication and talk therapy. Though none of these treatments have been rigorously studied, there is some clinical evidence that they may be helpful, and other than the cost, they are at least not harmful.

FIVE
other
treatments

Some people report that the over-the-counter products St. John's wort and Sam-e help relieve the symptoms of depression, but there is not any significant scientific data to support this. And, of course, it goes without saying that if your child is taking either of these products along with psychotropic medication, your child's psychiatrist *must* know about it. St. John's wort in particular can interact negatively with antidepressants and it may decrease the effectiveness of oral contraceptives. Both of these supplements can have side effects, including dry mouth, dizziness, diarrhea, nausea, fatigue, increased sensitivity to sunlight and constipation.

Neurofeedback is an experimental therapy for treatment of depression. It is a specific form of biofeedback in which the patient retrains his brain waves based on information he receives from the therapist, who reads the patient's brain waves via electrodes attached to the patient's scalp. The thinking is that, because of the plasticity of the brain, when we retrain the brain waves, rewiring takes place, and new thinking is established. Studies are currently underway to assess the efficacy and safety of neurofeedback.

ECT therapy (electroconvulsive therapy) is sometimes used to interrupt a severe case of depression or bipolar disorder, generally when other treatments have not been effective. In ECT, electrical currents are passed through the brain. Treatment consists of sessions a few times a week for between two and four weeks. Side effects can include immediate confusion after treatment and memory loss during the weeks of treatment.

Transcranial magnetic stimulation (TMS or rTMS) is an experimental treatment in which a magnetic field is used to provide electrical stimulation to the brain. It is typically used for people with depression who have not responded to other treatments, and sometimes is used instead of ECT.

Vagus (or Vagal) Nerve Stimulation—VNS—is another treatment that is sometimes used when other treatments have not worked. This treatment involves implanting a pacemaker-like device in the patient's chest and connecting the device via wiring to the vagus nerve located at the base of the brain. VNS has been approved by the FDA for treatment of depression in patients 18 years and older who have long-term, severe or recurrent depression that has not responded to other treatments. Research about its effectiveness is mixed.

And, as we all know, you will find many other alternative treatments by even a quick search of the Internet. As we said before, some of these treatments may be tempting. We can only say that it's important to talk to your child's physician and therapist before trying alternative treatments to make sure they are not harmful, especially if your child is taking psychotropic medication.

In addition, be wary of quick fixes—they are likely not supported by research, and may even be scams. It's wise to thoroughly research any alternative you want to try—we have a variety of websites listed at the back of the book which can give you an impartial description of the treatment and tell you whether there is sufficient evidence to support its use.

happiness

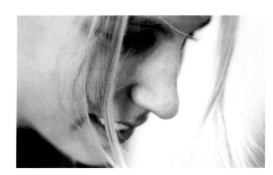

There is now a group of psychologists who are studying, not mental illness, but mental health—their research asks the question: **what does it take to make one happy?** Their answer? Three things:

- Strong, meaningful relationships
- A purpose to one's life
- Setting and achieving goals towards that purpose.

In their very simplicity, there is much to contemplate.

Though our handbook has been about depression and how to deal with it if your child is suffering from it, in some ways this handbook relates to the question of happiness. The underlying intention of the book is the same intention we give every day to raising our children—not just providing them with food, clothing and shelter, but providing them with a firm basis on which to stand as adults and achieve their own happiness.

As you travel the road that many of us have been down before, keep in mind that your ultimate goal is this goal too—the happiness of your child—and that it's the goal of every single parent, from time immemorial to the present second and beyond. We are all connected to one another in this very meaningful endeavor.

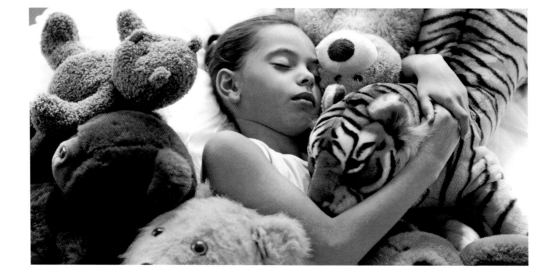

A CONCLUDING LETTER

We hope that this handbook has been useful to you. We know there are many more subjects we could have discussed in our handbook—when and how to find a therapeutic school for your child, what to do if your child requires hospitalization, etc. These are complicated issues, and we felt that they required more detailed explanations than we could give room to in this handbook. At some future date, we hope to provide this information on our website, *erikaslighthouse.org*.

It has been said that it takes a village to raise a child, and this handbook is our attempt to be a virtual village for you, to help at a particularly difficult time in your lives—a time when you might feel like there is no village out there for you.

If you need more information, there are many websites available on the Internet, and some good reference books available for purchase or at your local library. We have included those that we found particularly useful at the end of our handbook.

And while we've tried to be as accurate, complete and objective as we could in our handbook, please remember that we are parents—not professionals dispensing either medical or psychological advice. You should rely on your child's professionals for that.

We wish you and your family all the best. We welcome your comments and suggestions Please write to us at Post Office Box 616, Winnetka, Illinois 60093 or email us at *info@erikaslighthouse.org*.

> Sincerely,
> The Board of Directors
> Erika's Lighthouse
> March 2009

Pay it forward, pass it on … Just as we are passing this information along to you, we hope you will do the same. If you have a friend or neighbor in need of this handbook, please tell her that she can get a copy by sending an email to us or by downloading a copy from our website. And … thank you.

A LISTING OF MENTAL HEALTH SOCIAL SERVICE AGENCIES AND CLINICS IN THE NORTHERN SUBURBS OF CHICAGO

appendix

THE FAMILY INSTITUTE OF NORTHWESTERN UNIVERSITY
www.family-institute.org

Location:	Evanston (847) 733-4300
Counseling:	Yes
Assessments:	Yes
Referrals:	To Family Institute therapists
Ages served:	Adolescents through adults
Fee:	Sliding scale for clinic; hourly rates for individual therapists

FAMILY SERVICE OF GLENCOE
www.familyserviceofglencoe.org

Location:	Glencoe (847) 835-5111
Counseling:	Yes
Assessments:	No
Referrals:	Yes
Ages served:	All ages
Fee:	Sliding scale, no one is refused

FAMILY SERVICE OF WINNETKA-NORTHFIELD
www.familyservicewn.org

Location:	Winnetka (847) 446-8060
Counseling:	Yes
Assessments:	No
Referrals:	Yes
Ages served:	All ages
Fee:	Sliding scale, no one is refused

FAMILY SERVICE CENTER OF GLENVIEW/KENILWORTH/ NORTHBROOK/WILMETTE
www.familyservicecenter.com

Locations:	Glenview, Northbrook and Wilmette (847) 251-7350
Counseling:	Yes
Assessments:	No
Referrals:	Yes
Ages served:	All ages
Fee:	Sliding scale, accepts insurance, no one is refused

FAMILY SERVICE OF SOUTH LAKE COUNTY
www.fsslc.org

Location:	Highland Park (847) 432-4981
Counseling:	Yes
Assessments:	No
Referrals:	Yes
Ages served:	Ages 12 and over
Fee:	Sliding scale

HAVEN YOUTH AND FAMILY SERVICES
www.havenforyouth.org

Location:	Winnetka (847) 446-5606
Counseling:	Yes
Assessments:	No
Referrals:	Yes
Ages served:	Ages 12 through 18 and their families
Fee:	Free

METROPOLITAN FAMILY SERVICES
www.metrofamily.org

Locations:	Evanston and Skokie (847) 425-7400
Counseling:	Yes
Assessments:	Yes, but must get treatment there
Referrals:	Yes
Ages served:	All ages
Fee:	Variable—standard and sliding scale

YOU
www.youevanston.org

Location:	Evanston (847) 866-1200
Counseling:	Yes
Assessments:	No
Referrals:	Yes
Ages served:	All ages
Fee:	Free

JEWISH CHILD AND FAMILY SERVICES
www.jcfs.org

Locations:	Skokie (847) 568-5100
	Northbrook (847) 412-4350
	Arlington Heights (847) 392-8820
Counseling:	Yes
Assessments:	Yes
Referrals:	Yes
Ages served:	All ages
Fee:	Sliding scale

SAMARITAN COUNSELING CENTER
www.northshoresamaritan.org

Location:	Winnetka (847) 446-6955
Counseling:	Yes
Assessments:	No
Referrals:	Yes
Ages served:	All ages
Fee:	Sliding scale, no one is refused

YOUTH SERVICES OF GLENVIEW-NORTHBROOK
www.youthservices-gn.org

Location:	Glenview (847) 724-2620
Counseling:	Yes
Assessments:	No
Referrals:	Yes
Ages served:	Infant through 18 years old
Fee:	Fixed rates, no one is refused

JOSSELYN CENTER
www.josselyn.org

Location:	Northfield (847) 441-5600
Counseling:	Yes
Assessments:	Yes
Referrals:	Yes
Ages served:	All ages
Fee:	Sliding scale, accepts insurance, no one is refused

TURNING POINT
www.tpoint.org

Location:	Skokie (847) 933-0051
Counseling:	Yes
Assessments:	Yes
Referrals:	Yes
Ages served:	All ages
Fee:	Sliding scale

references
and further reading

There are many resources about childhood and adolescent depression available—in the form of videos, books, websites and other publications. As we have throughout our handbook, we encourage you to be informed about your child's illness. Here are some resources that we have found useful while writing our handbook. We hope that you will find them helpful too.

BOOKS

Adolescent Depression: A Guide for Parents
Francis Mark Mondimore, M.D.
The Johns Hopkins University Press, 2002

Helping Your Teenager Beat Depression:
A Problem-Solving Approach for Families
Katharine Manassis, M.D. and
Anne Marie Levac, R.N., M.N.
Woodbine House, Inc., 2004

If Your Adolescent Has Depression
or Bipolar Disorder: An Essential Resource
for Parents
Dwight L. Evans, M.D. and
Linda Wasmer Andrews
Oxford University Press, 2005

Straight Talk about Psychiatric Medications
for Kids, Revised Edition
Timothy E. Wilens, M.D.
The Guilford Press, 2004

Understanding Teenage Depression:
A Guide to Diagnosis, Treatment
and Management
Maureen Empfield, M.D. and
Nicholas Bakalar
Henry Holt and Company LLC, 2001

OTHER PUBLICATIONS

Blueprint for Change: Research on Child
and Adolescent Mental Health
The National Advisory Mental Health
Council Workgroup on Child and
Adolescent Mental Health Intervention
Development and Deployment,
Washington, D.C., 2001

Choosing the Right Treatment:
What Families Need to Know about
Evidence-Based Practices
The National Alliance on Mental Illness,
Arlington, VA, 2007

Medications, with Addendum January 2007
National Institute of Mental Health,
National Institutes of Health,
Bethesda, MD, 2002, 2007
NIH Publication No. 02-3929
http://www.nimh.nih.gov/health/
publications/medications/summary.shtml

Mental Health: A Report
of the Surgeon General
Substance Abuse and Mental Health
Services Administration, Center for Mental
Health Services, National Institute of Mental
Health, National Institutes of Health,
Rockville, MD, 1999
http://www.surgeongeneral.gov/library/
mentalhealth/home.html

Report of the Working Group on
Psychotropic Medications for Children
and Adolescents: Psychopharmacological,
Psychosocial, and Combined Interventions
for Childhood Disorders: Evidence Base,
Contextual Factors, and Future Directions
American Psychological Association,
Washington, D.C., 2006
http://www.apa.org/pi/cyf/childmeds.pdf

WEBSITES

The American Academy of Child
and Adolescent Psychiatry
www.aacap.org

The American Psychological Association
www.apa.org

Anxiety Disorders Association of America
www.adaa.org

The Child and Adolescent Bipolar Foundation
www.bpkids.org

Children and Adults with
Attention Deficit-Hyperactivity Disorder
www.chadd.org

Clinicaltrials.gov

Copecaredeal.org

The Depression and Bipolar Support Alliance
www.dbsalliance.org

Drugs.com

Families for Depression Awareness
www.familyaware.org

The Food and Drug Administration
www.fda.gov

Healthfinder.gov

Mayoclinic.com

Medlineplus.gov

Mental Health America
www.nmha.org

Narsad.org

The National Alliance on Mental Illness
www.nami.org

The National Association of Social Workers
www.socialworkers.org

National Eating Disorders Association
www.nationaleatingdisorders.org

The National Institute of Mental Health
www.nimh.nih.gov

Obsessive-Compulsive Foundation
www.ocfoundation.org

Pdrhealth.com

Psychcentral.com

VIDEOS

Frontline: "Inside the Teenage Brain"
Sarah Spinks
Frontline and PBS, 2002

Frontline: "The Medicated Child"
Marcela Gaviria
Frontline and PBS, 2008

about the authors

This book was a collaboration of many people over the course of a few years. The genesis of the book was a few brave parents sitting in a living room for many Wednesday afternoons, talking about what had happened to them and their children when confronted with an episode of depression. Those sessions gave us the beginning kernels of our collective wisdom—what worked and what didn't—and from those kernels, the handbook was born. Then, lots of research and reading books and studies about depression and treatment options ensued, along with interviews of professionals in our schools and the mental health community to gain the benefit of their expertise.

A final reading by parents and friends ironed out the wrinkles. It was a work of goodwill and countless hours spent on the part of many, who we thank and honor here:

Elaine Tinberg
Author

Karen Miller
Designer

Virginia Neuckranz
Founder and President
Erika's Lighthouse

Thomas H. Neuckranz
Founder
Erika's Lighthouse

Peggy G. Kubert, A.M., L.C.S.W.
Executive Director

Heather Steward
Teen Coordinator

Andy Robins
Youth Outreach

Cate Barron

Gwendolyn Britt

Kitsy Bryant, R.N.
School Nurse, retired

David C. Clark, Ph.D.

Matthew D. Cohen, Esq.

Craig Colmar

Nancy W. Condon, M.D.

Dianna Devine

Mark Ditthardt
Director of Pupil Services
Winnetka Public Schools

Mina K. Dulcan, M.D.
*Head of Child and
Adolescent Psychiatry*
Feinberg School of Medicine
at Northwestern University
Children's Memorial Hospital

Julia Jergensen Edelman

Mary Halpin, Ph.D.
School Psychologist
Washburne Middle School

Eileen Sheehan Hovey

Judith Bultman Meyer

JoAnn Olsen, M.D.

Melissa B. Perrin, Psy.D.

Dorit Raviv, Ph.D.

Tali Raviv, Ph.D.

Alec Ross, L.C.S.W.

Dan Schwartz, Ed.D.
Principal of Washburne School
Winnetka Public Schools

Kathleen Kelly Spear

Maggie Stewart

Barbara Bruck Williams

ERIKA'S LIGHTHOUSE

about Erika

Erika was a bright light who, sadly, lost her battle with depression in 2004 at age 14. She is missed and was much loved. Erika's Lighthouse was founded in her honor and is dedicated to helping other young people who struggle with depression.

TO REQUEST ADDITIONAL PRINTED COPIES of the *Parent Handbook on Childhood and Adolescent Depression* or to join our mailing list for news and information about Erika's Lighthouse, please go to *www.erikaslighthouse.org/contact/* or email us at *info@erikaslighthouse.org*.

TO DOWNLOAD A COPY of the *Parent Handbook on Childhood and Adolescent Depression*, please go to *www.erikaslighthouse.org*.

TO MAKE A TAX-DEDUCTIBLE DONATION to Erika's Lighthouse, please go to *www.erikaslighthouse.org/donate/* or make your check payable to Erika's Lighthouse and mail it to us at Erika's Lighthouse, Post Office Box 616, Winnetka, Illinois 60093. Thank you!